The reality of mental illness

The reality of mental illness

MARTIN ROTH & JEROME KROLL

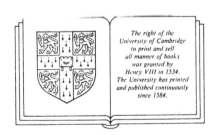

The right of the
University of Cambridge
to print and sell
all manner of books
was granted by
Henry VIII in 1534.
The University has printed
and published continuously
since 1584.

CAMBRIDGE UNIVERSITY PRESS

Cambridge
London New York New Rochelle
Melbourne Sydney

CAMBRIDGE UNIVERSITY PRESS
Cambridge, New York, Melbourne, Madrid, Cape Town, Singapore, São Paulo, Delhi

Cambridge University Press
The Edinburgh Building, Cambridge CB2 8RU, UK

Published in the United States of America by Cambridge University Press, New York

www.cambridge.org
Information on this title: www.cambridge.org/9780521337618

First published 1986
Re-issued in this digitally printed version 2009

A catalogue record for this publication is available from the British Library

Library of Congress Cataloguing in Publication data
Roth, Martin, 1917–
The reality of mental illness.
1. Psychiatry – Philosophy.   2. Mental illness – Etiology.
I. Kroll, Jerome.   II. Title.
RC437.5.R68   1986   616.89   85-29935

ISBN 978-0-521-32151-8 hardback
ISBN 978-0-521-33761-8 paperback

For Constance and Kathleen

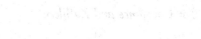

Contents

Acknowledgements

The authors would like to thank Ms Kris Servin and Ms Jill Nagorski for their patient typing of the many revisions of this manuscript, and to express their appreciation to their colleagues who have read and generously offered critiques of the manuscript: from the University of Minnesota, Professor Bernard Bachrach, Department of History; Professor Leonard Heston, Department of Psychiatry; Professor Robert Levy, School of Law; Professor Michael Root, Department of Philosophy; from Cornell University Medical College, Professor Jacques Quen, Department of Psychiatry; also the late Professor Karl Britton and Professor Anthony Whitlock.

Introduction

It would be advantageous if one could offer the reader an uncomplicated description of psychiatry. This would encompass a description of its subject matter (mental illness), methods and goals (diagnosis, treatment, research and prevention). The ideal of such a presentation, however, appears unrealistic for two main reasons. First the descriptions and causes of aberrations of human behaviour, which constitute the subject matter of psychiatry, are themselves extremely complicated and therefore require cautious hypotheses and statements rather than pretentious assertions. Second, many of the working hypotheses, methods and goals of psychiatry are presently under attack, and these criticisms require an answer. The charges against psychiatry include the following: that mental illnesses are merely socially deviant behaviours rather than real illnesses; that medicine has traditionally been disinterested in mental illnesses until about two hundred years ago when it became apparent that profit was to be had in taking charge of asylums and their inmates; that in Western industrialized societies psychiatrists serve their capitalist masters by defining as mentally ill and confining in mental hospitals those who are social dissenters, troublemakers, and economically unproductive; that mental illnesses are created by psychiatrists by the very act of diagnosis; and that mental illness, if it exists at all, should not provide an excuse for criminal behaviour or a justification for involuntary hospitalization.

This book will attempt to describe the complex field of psychiatry and the many ethical, social and scientific problems that arise as human beings interact with one another. It will at the same time consider the charges of psychiatry's critics as these charges appear relevant to the particular topic being discussed.

We will begin by offering examples of mentally ill persons as they come to the attention of their families and communities, and eventually of psychiatrists. To the ordinary person, these examples speak persuasively as familiar forms of suffering for which medical care has appeared indispensable. We will proceed in Chapters 2 and 3 to demonstrate that, since the beginnings of written history, society has recognized mental illnesses and has expected medicine as a profession to accept responsibility for treating such problems. Further, it will be seen that the major characteristics, familiar to the general public, of symptomatic psychoses, schizophrenia and manic-depressive illnesses have been clearly recognized with some variations in every culture submitted to enquiry.

We will demonstrate in Chapters 4 and 5 that the concepts of illness and disease are *not* to be regarded as all or none constructs permitting axiomatic definitions devoid of all ambiguity. Indeed, a quest for pinning down with complete precision the meaning of such terms is a form, to use Popper's phrase, of empty verbalism. Our concepts of illness and disease are hypotheses, in some cases thousands of years old, about the nature of various forms of suffering, and are still in the process of being formulated and refined. We hope to substantiate the position that concepts of illness as used by psychiatrists do not differ from the use of such concepts by other medical practitioners. All concepts of disease begin as descriptions of behavioural states, with causes unknown. It is the diligent description of such illnesses which provides the indispensable precondition for the development of theories of disease, the testing of these theories against additional observations, and the consequent increase in knowledge.

This method of medical classification, which in the realm of psychiatry is attacked by critics as dehumanizing and destructive, has in fact been of immeasurable benefit to human well-being. The contributions of the psychodynamic and pharmacological approaches to the understanding and treatment of mental illnesses were born of direct observations in the clinic which were accumulated in various combinations until meaningful patterns could be discovered. We hope to make it clear that the concept of disease is wider in practice than the concrete examples of 'diseases' advanced by critics of psychiatry who insist upon the presence of structural pathology, and incorporates sociological and psychological factors. Thus not only conditions with demonstrable physical pathology in specific organs, such as pneumonia, brain tumours or broken arms, can be considered diseases, but so too can conditions demonstrating altered function, such as hypertension, diabetes, asthma, schizophrenia and anorexia nervosa.

Finally, with respect to both ancient and recent medical-legal issues, we examine in Chapter 6 situations that pose painful dilemmas to medicine, society, to the individuals affected by mental illnesses and their families. Epidemiological and clinical studies have repeatedly demonstrated that there is an increased mortality from psychiatric disorders not only as a result of suicide but also from increased morbidity of other illnesses. For example, the increased death rates in cases of cancer complicated by depression, of markedly anxious patients who have had a myocardial infarction compared with emotionally undisturbed heart patients, and of cardiac surgery patients who express hopelessness and wishes for death at the time of surgery all demonstrate the increased risk which untreated psychiatric disorders, especially depression, bring to the patient.

In addition, the antipsychiatry writers often ignore the very tangible devastation which mental illness imposes upon patients and their family. Job loss, family disruption, economic hardship, loss of educational opportunities, and social drift downwards are all frequent consequences, rather than causes, of serious mental illness. A significant part of this suffering and loss can be prevented with readily available pharmacological and psychological treatments.

Furthermore, although the majority of people with serious mental illnesses are not dangerous, there is a substantial minority whose conduct places the community at grave risk. In some cases the correlations are well known, as in the risk of spouse murder by persons with morbid jealousy or the sexual offenders who employ violence in the execution of their crimes. The dangerous psychopath also represents one of the most controversial medical-legal issues, namely the question of whether character disorders should be accorded illness-status. It is problematic how far such disorders are predetermined by genetic and developmental influences in the formative years, and to what extent such unwelcome influences should mitigate responsibility.

There is a dilemma here for all societies that have attained and strive to live by civilized standards. It is implicit in human relationships within such societies that individuals are responsible for their actions. Yet they know them to be shaped and to function within certain limits by heredity and by the vicissitudes of the early formative years. The laws which hold people responsible are not peculiar to any one kind of political system or social organization. They are an indispensable precondition for the establishment of trusting human relationships and for the creation of communities whose citizens can be vouchsafed an adequate measure of security and protection. For this reason those who flagrantly break such rules are made to suffer disapproval or punishment. The more extreme forms of rule-breaking are regarded as crimes and certain types of crime, for example, the predatory murder of strangers is execrated and condemned in all cultures. But exceptions to such implicit rules have been made since the beginning of recorded history. Most societies have recognized diminished responsibility of individuals with certain forms of mental disorder while striving at the same time to protect its citizens. Such exceptions have been judged essential in the interests of compassion and justice.

Psychiatry and the behavioural sciences have played a part in describing a socio-medical profile of psychopathic personality disorders, but have been less successful in changing them. The question of whether psychological medicine should remain involved in the diagnosis, treatment and assessment of risk of these disorders is a problem of immense complexity. We discuss both sides of the issue in Chapter 6. We see a need to strike a fair and equitable balance between the requirements of society for protection and justice and the rights of the individual.

It has been the traditional role of the medical sciences to soften harsh moralistic ideas and punitive attitudes that have prevailed historically. With regard to homosexuality and other behaviours that have often been defined by law as misdemeanours, science has brought a more objective and compassionate approach by arguing that deviance is not due to original sin but stems from the influence of early factors. The advance of science has helped societies in their thinking about aberrant behaviours to move from moralistic-theistic concepts to definable naturalistic mechanisms that may ultimately be either alterable or acceptable as legitimate alternatives. In the case of the behaviour disorders, we run into serious philosophical and social problems. We discuss these problems in Chapter 6 also, and offer tentative approaches rather than final, simplistic, absolute solutions.

We judge it essential to spell out to the reader certain *caveats* regarding the generalizations which we employ and to ensure that the many qualifications and nuances which might otherwise be lost are at least acknowledged. Thinking and writing in our culture traditionally follow a linear progression and therefore automatically and immediately do an injustice to the richness of most complex subject matters. In a consideration of human behaviours within a biological and social context, many events and analyses are occurring simultaneously, and contradictory and complementary attitudes exist side by side. Words, however, can only be placed one alongside the other. Consequently, while one statement is presented – such as 'the biological model has replaced the psychological model as the dominant aetiological hypothesis regarding mental illness' – all the other statements which might half-contradict this one or which might suggest the numerous nuances which must be attached to the core statement in order to make it a thoughtful premise which accurately reflects *all* the complexities attached to it, must patiently wait as the ticker-tape of thought slowly unrolls. The problem is that every statement requires a footnote or a textual paragraph to clarify and correct it; yet repeated qualifications and caveats would be tedious and confusing. We therefore trust the reader will appreciate that there is an opposite side and multiple facets to every statement, that a dominant hypothesis does not wholly invalidate alternative hypotheses, and that small parcels of theory and data are constantly being attached to and extruded from the dominant theory.

1 Mental illness, psychiatry and its critics

At first thought, there does not seem to be any compelling reason why someone who behaves strangely, complains of hallucinatory voices, of enemies who pry into his intimate thoughts through the television screen, speaks incoherently and tries without cause to take his own life should be considered as having an illness. The word 'illness' conjures up diabetes, pneumonia, myocardial infarct and epilepsy, which appear to have little resemblance to conditions such as agoraphobia, schizophrenia and manic-depressive psychosis. The range of behaviour patterns and experiences to which the term mental illness is applied appears to merge with mere human eccentricities and even with normality itself.

On the other hand, the nature of the conditions regarded by psychiatrists as forms of 'mental illness' seem so clear and self-evident that one may puzzle why there should be any controversy at all. All societies throughout the ages have recognized the existence of insanity or mental illness among some of their members, and have distinguished these from conditions such as feeble-mindedness, criminality, and incongruent gender roles or sexual behaviour. It is true that near the boundaries between mental illness and criminality, feeble-mindedness, and even normality the distinction can be hard to make. Such difficulties, however, have not prevented all societies from recognizing and providing special care for sufferers from those conditions identical with the forms of mental suffering which within our own culture are denoted as mental disorders. Furthermore, the indigenous descriptions of mental illness within very disparate cultures are extraordinarily similar and demonstrate the repetition of a few basic elements: incoherent speech, bizarre and idiosyncratic beliefs, purposeless or unpredictable or violent behaviour, and apparent absence of concern for one's own safety and comfort. These features appear to be universal, across time and geography.

Basic questions regarding human behaviour

These, then, are the two crucial issues. First, how does it come about that certain types of behaviour and experience are regarded as illnesses? Is there justification for this position by an examination of the facts of nature rather than by an appeal to the labelling havits of different cultures? Second, in the face of a universal and immediate experience of certain types of mental illness, how does it happen that

5

a small number of influential writers claim that there is no such thing; that those persons who appear to suffer from any of these conditions are merely adapting their behaviours to conform with the labels of deviancy that are applied to them; that special concessions and rules ought not to be granted to those who appear to be 'insane'; and, since such conditions bear no relation to illness, those affected should not be cared for or treated by the medical profession?

The phenomena of mental illness evoke questions of great complexity for which dogmatic and simplistic answers do not exist. These questions involve the relationship of minds to bodies, the nature of human motivation, the real or illusory nature of free will as against predetermined action, and the puzzle of human illness seemingly both mental and physical. It is in the field of medicine in general, and psychiatry in particular, that our deepest philosophical questions and disagreements about human obligations, values and responsibilities become concrete. Society is forced to move from thinking about abstract principles to the making of hard choices – decisions about involuntary hospitalization, the administration of medication and other treatments with a risk of harmful side-effects, decisions about criminal responsibility. And each one of these choices may profoundly affect the lives of those persons who are subjected to them. The institutions of government – courts of law, legislatures – must determine how far it is justifiable to interfere with personal autonomy in the interests of society. It is, no doubt, the nature of the ordinary world that complicated problems are ultimately reduced to and resolved by yes/no decisions: to medicate or not medicate, hospitalize or not hospitalize. But pragmatically reducing a knotty problem to a simple solution does not mean that the issues are ever clear or that boundaries are unambiguous. The decisions required of us may be agonizingly difficult; it does not serve either society or the physician well to pretend otherwise.

Some examples of mental illness

To bring the subject sharply into focus, it may be helpful to consider a few brief accounts of the development of states of mind which caused those affected to be thought of as 'mentally ill'. It was rarely psychiatrists who first formed this opinion. Spouses, parents, friends, relatives and, in some cases, members of the public had reached the same conclusion. The attachment of a psychiatric diagnosis or label, or time spent in a mental hospital, were not the causes of the disturbed behaviour or the concomitant mental distress. These had been manifest previously. The influence of newspapers, television and other media in shaping people's attitudes may also be discounted. For, as we plan to establish, the states of mind to be described are very similar to those in descriptions handed down through the centuries, from the beginnings of recorded history.

Case 1

A married woman of 50 had previously suffered a depressive illness of five months' duration when she was aged 37. The day before the present admission to the psychiatric unit of a university hospital her 21-year-old son had been stabbed to death a few yards from her home. Her immediate response when she learned the news was to run lamenting and screaming into the street, tearing her hair, pounding her head and body and lacerating her face and neck. This behaviour settled within a few hours of admission and there followed a half-day during which she was quiet, immobile and unresponsive. She then became suddenly over-active, continuously moving around the ward, shifting the furniture, taking the possessions of others and scattering them around the ward. She burst into rapid, voluble and excited speech with an abundance of rhymes, puns, jokes and obscene words wholly out of character for her. She was excited, distracted, sang songs in endless succession and made jocular remarks about the staff and patients and displayed disinhibited erotic behaviour. She appeared wholly oblivious of her son's death. She was awake at 5.00 a.m. and began the day writing ten- to twenty-page letters to the Queen, members of the Royal family, the prime minister and local dignitaries.

After two weeks in the hospital the state of acute elation was interrupted by brief episodes of agitated depression in which she exhibited the previous pattern of grieving, lamenting and tearing her flesh. She moaned and bewailed her son's fate and blamed herself for neglecting to care for him. She was actively suicidal and had to be restrained to prevent her from plunging a knife into her chest or hurling herself through a window. Such brief surges of acute depression were abruptly interrupted by a recrudescence of her manic state which predominated during this phase of her illness. She was treated psychologically by means of the relationship established with doctors and nurses and with a combination of antipsychotic medication and lithium carbonate. She gradually became more subdued over a period of three weeks. Her condition then settled into a state of mute retarded depression in which it was difficult to get her to eat or drink. With the aid of antidepressive treatment she gradually improved over the next four weeks. Three months after admission she had returned to her normal self and though continuing to mourn her son, was able to return home and function effectively in the roles of wife and mother and to perform her domestic duties.

She was much concerned about her relapse after a twelve-year interval of healthy life and was distressed by memories of the pattern of behaviour during the early manic phases of her illness. She had not experienced manic symptoms during her previous illness. She was worried also about a possible recrudescence of what she regarded as a serious illness and was anxious to be treated and supervised so as to minimize the chances of relapse.

During the first five weeks of illness following her bereavement a state of paradoxical elation predominated in this woman's mental state, interrupted by brief surges of intense depression. She was diagnosed and treated for a manic-depressive illness and it is doubtful whether any other view of her condition could have saved her from taking her life.

Case 2

A girl of 18 became mildly depressed after learning that her performance in a recent examination had been disappointing. Ten weeks later she left with her parents and grandparents for a holiday in France. She remained despondent and a little taciturn but was able to cheer up in the presence of congenial company. A week after arriving in Paris she developed the idea that after the first encounter with one of her French relatives there had been a change in her body and she wondered whether she was becoming a man. For several days in succession she experienced the hallucination of having sexual intercourse with her uncle who lived in another French town 300 miles away. She was observed to carry out rhythmic bodily movements followed by outbursts of shouting, screaming and weeping. She complained that her behaviour was being relayed by television to all her friends and relatives in England.

She thought that the actions of people around her implied that she should kill herself and she heard the voice of God ordering her to die. When other people looked at her she experienced further sensations of bodily changes towards a more masculine physique. Every action by others and every tick of the clock appeared to have some sinister and mysterious significance she could not fathom. The world appeared unfamiliar, alien and permeated by some evil force. All remarks made to her seemed to carry a double meaning. She wore a look of perplexity and bewilderment. Twelve days after leaving England she was stuporous and mute and was admitted to a mental hospital. In a sudden bout of agitation she tried to throw herself out of a window. She explained subsequently that in attempting suicide she was seeking to escape from the ever-present conviction that she could kill others by glancing at them.

She made a good response to pharmacological treatment and supportive psychotherapy. However, there was some adverse change from her previous cheerful, bouncy and outgoing personality to being withdrawn emotionally, cold and unresponsive, apathetic, lacking in initiative and curiosity. She was fearful of watching television because all communications seemed to refer to her.

This girl's illness had indeed followed partial failure in an examination and some minor difficulties in her relationship with her boyfriend. But these were mere hand-claps which brought down an avalanche. She was judged to be suffering from a schizophrenic illness from which she made a partial recovery following treatment and rehabilitation. She is able to work as a clerk on a part-time basis.

We have begun with examples of psychiatric illness which provide a clear and, in our view, indubitable starting point for its definition. It need hardly be emphasized that, as is the case with all concepts developed from observation of the real world, the boundaries and limits cannot be drawn in clear and sharp lines.

There is, for example, place for debate regarding the dividing line between normal behaviour and neurotic states. But even in this territory, certain disorders are found in which a kinship with medical disease may be postulated. At the very least a disease hypothesis seems as justified as any other formulation and has in many cases already proved of practical value. Two examples of neurotic disorders must suffice.

Case 3
A 33-year-old married woman discovered some beetles while clearing out an old cupboard in her house. She immediately had to wash her hands and to repeat the washing three times. Each time she cleaned or dusted the house she began to wash her hands three times, and thereafter in increasing multiples of three. She was soon washing her hands hundreds of times a day and thereafter felt compelled to bathe herself between six and nine times daily. All the time she recognized that these compulsions were morbid but felt helpless against them. In the next stage of the disorder she developed the belief that every object that might have come into contact with hair had become contaminated. She began to dispose of her own and her husband's personal possessions and thereafter to sell articles of furniture ridiculously cheaply. At the time of her admission, an entire suite of furniture from her house had been sold and the patient came in covered by an unused bedsheet, the only uncontaminated object in the home that could be used to cover her naked body. She made a good response to treatment with pharmacological and behavioural methods and psychotherapy and returned home with minimal symptoms after ten weeks in the hospital.

Case 4

An 18-year-old girl who had recently begun a degree course at university thought herself to be obese, ugly and ungainly in comparison with other women students in her class. She began to avoid all carbohydrate food and her weight declined from 47.7 kilograms (105 lb) to 38.2 kilograms (84 lb) during her first year. Towards the end of the year she began to indulge in binges after dinner, eating a loaf of bread, or half a tin of biscuits or a cake or a box of chocolates. Abnormal distension and discomfort and intense feelings of guilt followed such bouts of over-eating which were often terminated by self-induced vomiting. Her weight began to show marked fluctuations of 3.5–5.0 kilograms (8–10 lb) from one month to the next. Intense depression, guilt and suicidal urges were regular concomitants of periods in which she gained weight. She came under psychiatric observations following a serious suicidal attempt in which she swallowed one hundred aspirin tablets she had bought at a pharmacist. She had to be resuscitated in an intensive care unit.

What constitutes disease?

Critics of psychiatry would regard these examples of mental suffering as descriptions of non-illness or social protest. They would further regard the psychiatric approach to them as forms of mystification in which veiled account is taken of social and moral problems and the whole result manipulated for the maintenance and protection of the established order. It is difficult to categorize the critics of psychiatry, because the different critics disagree with each other in some areas and overlap in others. Fundamentally, criticisms against psychiatry seem to fall into two major groupings. The first consists of those who assert that there are no such things as mental illnesses. Within this group, one subgroup, represented by Thomas Szasz, explains the seeming presence of persons with mental illness by asserting that most of them are frauds, mere simulators of craziness.[1] Another subgroup, represented by Lemert, Goffman, Scheff and Rosenhan, claims that persons begin to act as though mentally ill only after and as a result of having been labelled as such by psychiatrists acting as agents of the dominant social order.[2] Members of the second major grouping of critics of psychiatry, unlike the first, acknowledge to greater or lesser degrees that there are such things as mental illnesses, or rather, that persons do indeed become mentally ill. They claim, however, that mental illnesses are not diseases in the medical sense, but are reactions to unbearable stresses in life. This approach is represented by R. D. Laing, who lays the blame for mental illnesses upon the tyrannical bourgeois family which drives sensitive, creative souls into schizophrenia as their only escape from the madness of the ordinary world.[3] Another subgroup agrees somewhat with Laing, but broadens the attack by blaming the capitalist structure of society for causing the great misery which is acted out as mental illness. Representatives of this approach are Foucault and Basaglia.[4]

One criticism that occupies a place of central importance in this attack on the concept of mental illness is that persons exhibiting these states of mind do not have demonstrable evidence of damage to the body, that is, physical lesions or signs of infection or other pathology. Let us trace the implications of such an argument. One hundred and fifty years ago there was no knowledge of lesions present in conditions now universally regarded as being diseases. The underlying neurological basis of epilepsy had not been discovered. It was widely believed to be a disease of the mind and was described as such in textbooks of psychiatry. Similarly, paralysis agitans (Parkinson's disease) was considered by Charcot to develop from the 'violent moral emotions' aroused by the political unrest prevalent in France in 1877. It would have been false, according to such a view, to say that persons suffering from Parkinson's disease had *any* disease whatsoever – that is, false between 1817, when Parkinson initially described the clinical syndrome, and 1914 when Lewy elucidated the pathological anatomy of the basal ganglia of the brain in Parkinson's disease.[5] Farrell remarks on the absurdity of such thinking that, should our present views about its brain pathology prove to be false, then persons with paralysis agitans would once again be said to have no disease.[6]

Until the nineteenth century no lesions had been discerned as such in the majority of individuals we now recognize as suffering from specific endocrine disorders, such as diabetes or adrenal insufficiency. Before radiology came upon the scene the commonest forms of abdominal pain, discomfort and indigestion lacked any known physical causes. And even today a substantial proportion of patients in the care of gastroenterologists suffer from disorders lacking any known physical cause. 'Functional dyspepsia' or 'spastic colon' is hypothesized, but a physical basis is rarely demonstrated. An emotional cause is suspected by some physicians and a subtle form of physiological dysfunction by others. These are non-illnesses and non-diseases by the criteria of the critics of psychiatry. But those afflicted are unable to work, to function normally as spouses, parents and members of society and their sufferings are extreme.

Non-diseases, serious and fatal

One hundred and fifty years ago, mental hospitals were filled to a great extent by patients with a variety of conditions that we now know are caused by physical lesions. These include delirious states caused by infectious, metabolic and toxic illnesses that could not be diagnosed, such as the advanced syphilitic condition general paralysis of the insane, for which no specific diagnosis could be made in the early stages of the infection for lack of known physical signs. There must have been occasional patients with tumours of the temporal and frontal lobes and states of cerebral degeneration in conditions such as Alzheimer's disease and chronic subdural haematoma which were unidentified and undiagnosed at the time. General paralysis was generally attributed to moral turpitude and sexual excess – on the basis of social and ethical criteria and not medical ones. In short, 150 years ago there were virtually no diseases the lesions or physical causes of which could be established in life, and few were discovered after death. Accordingly, 'disease' as understood by the criteria of Szasz and many sociologists who follow in his wake, was very rare. But 'non-diseases', manifest in great mental and physical suffering and causing premature death in childhood and early adulthood, were very common.

There are other complex issues ignored or suppressed by this argument. A progression which is the reverse of what we have described may occur in relation to a 'disease'. Conditions attributed to physical causes in one generation, and seemingly qualifying as authentic diseases, may be shown in the next generation to have no such physical foundation. 'Anorexia nervosa', or 'bulimia nervosa' as some forms are described at the present time, was attributed until about half a century ago to a lesion of the anterior pituitary gland. Textbooks of medicine and physiology were illustrated forty or fifty years ago by memorable photographs of women in a state of advanced cachexia looking like survivors of Auschwitz or Belsen. We now know that there is no pituitary disease or even primary dysfunction of the gland. Young people who suffer from anorexia nervosa qualify for recognition as patients with a disease only on the basis of criteria identical with those that define depressive illness and schizophrenia. No physical causes are known and no lesions have been found.

The commonest mental disorders found among the aged provide further examples. Until three or four decades ago most forms of disturbed mental functioning beginning after the age of 60 were attributed to aging and the somatic and cerebral degenerative changes that accompany the aging process. At that time, then, such disorders would have been viewed by critics of psychiatry as cases of true 'disease'. But we have since realized that these concomitant physical changes are often insignificant and irrelevant in a broad range of behavioural disorders of the aged; identical changes can be found in mentally healthy persons of comparable age. Emotional illnesses dominated by anxiety or depression, neurotic conditions, paranoid psychoses and various forms of delirious states at first may appear as indistinguishable from progressive dementia; if properly diagnosed, however, they can now be treated successfully.[7] Somatic methods of treatment occupy an important, but not exclusive, role in the management of those affected. As a result of the discoveries that have opened the way for these advances in diagnosis and treatment, especially of depression, the functional impairments of cognition in the elderly have been relegated into the limbo of 'non-disease' by the criteria of psychiatry's critics.

There are other reasons why the criterion of demarcation between disease and non-disease on which critics of psychiatry insist is obfuscating and false. The strictures they have pronounced upon psychiatrists and their concepts, and their own delimitation of the realm of 'true disease', are opposite sides of the same coin. If illnesses were entirely confined to lesions of solid tissues, no emotional or familial factors would be relevant to the practice of medicine. This relegation of the physician to the role of a technician would lead to a dehumanized medicine divorced from all consideration of the personality-related and emotional concomitants observed in the majority of serious diseases of high mortality. It would be unacceptable to the medical profession and damaging and repugnant to the great majority of those who seek the help of doctors, even for what appear ostensibly to be purely somatic complaints.

If illness and disease consist of 'lumps, lesions and germs', what is the status of the conditions in which both physical and emotional factors have been shown to be contributory causes? Raised blood pressure, with its complications in cardiac failure, myocardial infarction and strokes, is caused to a considerable extent by genetic, physical and endocrine factors. But emotional stress and recurrent depression in particular have been shown to predispose to its development. The variation in the prevalence of hypertension in different countries, cultures, classes and ethnic groups is a related phenomenon.[8] Are such conditions in which definable and treatable affective disorder has been shown to contribute to the causation to be classed as 'disease' or 'non-disease'? And is the physician who concerns himself with the psychological and social aspects of such diseases to be judged as exceeding his proper role and encroaching upon individual and social prerogatives?

The complexity of these questions is further appreciated if we examine the interrelationships between 'diseases' and 'non-diseases' as defined by critics of psychiatry. On the one hand, those suffering from the most common psychiatric maladies, the affective and anxiety disorders, have been shown in clinical and epidemiological studies to have a significant excess of somatic illness as well as increased mortality rates.[9] But the clinical correlation also occurs in the opposite direction. A depressive illness is sometimes the earliest warning of a seemingly unrelated, non-neurological disease. A depression may affect patients who are completely unaware and unsuspecting of the presence of a significant physical disease such as a malignant growth.[10] It remains unclear whether such depressive disorders seen in association with occult physical lesions such as pancreatic carcinoma would qualify as 'disease' on the criteria of psychiatry's critics. And what of those schizophrenic syndromes developed in the context of amphetamine addiction?[11] Perhaps the physical condition (weight loss, rapid pulse) is 'disease' and the mental state (paranoid psychosis, racing thoughts) is 'non-disease'. It would then become difficult to understand why the treatment of physical disease and withdrawal of amphetamine should cause depressions to recede and some psychoses to abate.

To use the presence of physical lesions and lumps as the benchmark of demarcation of 'disease' from 'non-disease' is, accordingly, confused and misconceived. Only by a sleight of hand may the domain of conditions dealt with by physicians of every kind be neatly bisected in such a manner. Such conditions as schizophrenia, manic-depressive illness and obsessive compulsive disorders cannot be excluded from this domain. For as we shall attempt to demonstrate, the concept of 'mental disease' has proved of great value in the practice of medicine. It has advanced a set of testable hypotheses which have already borne fruit concerning the nature, causation and treatment of several of the very common and incapacitating forms of human suffering.

The implication of indefinite boundaries

Another reason advanced by critics who claim that 'mental illness' does not exist is the observation that the boundary line between normal and abnormal mental life is blurred. Anxieties, depressions, phobias and delusions merge imperceptibly with the ebb and flow of ordinary mental life. Yet the same vague, uncertain area between health and disease is present in relation to the commonest types of physical illness including diabetes, hypertension, respiratory disease, indigestion, epilepsy, headache, and intellectual impairment in old age. The observation that a concept has indefinite boundaries and that unequivocal judgements in all parts of the terrain to which it refers are not possible merely reflects the absence of sharp lines of demarcation in nature. Furthermore, a concept which has uncertain application in borderline cases may have a wide range of cases for which application is entirely beyond doubt. Even well-understood diseases within medicine may not be perfectly delineated by mathematical symbols or words for the purposes of making a decision in an individual case. In areas of uncertainty between health and disease the physician cannot afford to aim at immaculate diagnoses. His responsibility is to act wisely and to weigh the benefits of intervening with treatment against the dangers and hazards that may follow from it or against the possible consequences of no treatment. Those who assert that 'disease' has a clear and precise meaning in its application to the body but is devoid of all such significance when applied to the mind are wrong on both counts.

Explanations of mental disease from labelling theory

There are two additional variations of the argument that mental illnesses do not exist. The first asserts that psychiatric disorders are nothing more than the consequences of attaching an illness label to various behaviour patterns that deviate from conventional standards. A corollary of this theory holds that the full clinical picture and deteriorating course of illnesses such as schizophrenia are caused not by the unfolding of the disease process itself, but by the effects of hospitalization upon the person who was not ill at the time of hospitalization, but merely was a little deviant. Labelling theory holds that such 'primary deviance' falls within a normal state of mind and does not, in itself, cause any impediment or maladaptation for the individual concerned. The sufferings of patients begin, it is claimed, only when agents of society intervene – agents who have been specially trained to negate or silence deviance by defaming the deviant with a diagnosis of mental illness. Most members of society have been preconditioned to hold in contempt those so labelled and are prepared to have them incarcerated. It is further claimed that the application of the label and the stigma that attaches to it bring about disturbed behaviour.[12] But no evidence has been offered by antipsychiatrists to demonstrate that such a causal progression does indeed occur.

Two studies, by Gove[13] and van Praag,[14] critically examined the arguments put forth by the social labelling theorists and discovered either an absence of evidence or evidence that was contradictory to their assertions. Specifically, the social labelling theorists' major claim that the deviant behaviour is of minor consequence and practically unnoticed until a professional attaches an illness label is unequivocally contrary to the evidence. It has been demonstrated in several studies that families are painfully aware of the disturbed behaviour and mental state of their family member and have either tried to deny to themselves the serious nature of the illness or have sought to contain and conceal the psychotic person until the symptomatic behaviours became so alarming or protracted that they could no longer be ignored. Only then does the family seek medical attention for the ill member.[15] Only then, months to years after the onset and full development of the illness, is a psychiatric diagnosis offered. As Gove stated, 'It was found that hospitalization interrupted a situation which was experienced as untenable and, by doing so, it blocked actions which threatened irremediable damage to family life.'[16]

Furthermore the social labelling theorists ignore the manifest abnormality of much of the symptomatic behaviour, choosing instead to call it minor. They never explain why such primary *major* deviation occurs in the first place; rather they make light of it as eccentricities. In fact, most admissions to psychiatric hospitals are on a voluntary basis, with the person seeking admission to the hospital. Many patients who bring themselves to the hospital are not admitted because in the physician's judgement they are not impaired enough. The publicized image of the hospital gates opening wide to gobble up innocent and helpless eccentrics provides sensational copy for newspaper and television, but bears little relation to reality.

The question of whether institutionalization is sufficient to account for all or even most of the schizophrenic behaviours, such as hallucinations, delusions, incoherent thinking, social isolation and blunted emotions, is a critically important one. Goffman, who has been one of the most influential writers of this viewpoint, explains schizophrenic behaviour in a quaint, trivializing way that is characteristic of the 'double-bind' school that once sought to explain schizophrenia as an interpersonal gambit. Following admission, according to Goffman, the erstwhile non-ill person, now a patient, may 'avoid talking to anyone, may stay by himself when possible, and may even be "out of contact" or "manic" so as to avoid ratifying any interaction that presses a politely reciprocal role upon him'.[17]

We may compare this clever explanation offered by Goffman, which tells us much about Goffman's imaginativeness but little about schizophrenia, with the case of a young man we saw recently who had jumped off a high bridge in obedience to hallucinatory commands, and who was now ignoring us because he was still listening to the same voices.

Anyone who has worked (or spent time) in both a prison and a mental hospital will appreciate the fact that institutional life, however harsh or demoralizing, does not in itself cause schizophrenia. If it did, then the prisons would be filled with schizophrenics, which they most certainly are not. The difference is most clearly brought out by the realization that riots occur only in prisons, not in mental hospitals, although the low ratio of staff to patients in a dayroom of a mental ward could provide an ideal setting for a riot and a 'takeover'. The reason for this difference is relatively straightforward: schizophrenia as an illness leaves the patients socially withdrawn, emotionally blunted and disinterested in forming close or advantageous social bonds. This is a result of the illness, not of hospitalization, and is seen even in the young chronic schizophrenics who have never been hospitalized. By contrast, the inmates of a prison form social groups and protective and aggressive gangs: they lift weights, play cards, socialize and scheme together; they form committees to improve their situation and they engage in collaborative group action, including riots. If institutionalization created the schizophrenia-like picture of apathy, then prisoners and chronic schizophrenics would closely resemble each other after five to ten years of confinement.

If mental hospitals have been guilty, it has not been of causing schizophrenia, but rather of accepting a group of ill human beings who are specifically vulnerable to the demoralizing effects of a stagnant, unstimulating environment, and providing exactly that environment. But here we would hold society culpable, for establishing a priority system that assigns insufficient resources to the care of the mentally ill. Studies by Wing and Brown have clearly demonstrated that social deprivation increases symptoms of withdrawal and apathy, and that active rehabilitation programmes that are not overly intrusive bring about improvement in social behaviours, but not cures of schizophrenia.[18]

Rosenhan, in a related attack on the credibility of the way mental hospitals view patients, published a study in 1973 which reported that normal persons were admitted to psychiatric wards and were diagnosed as schizophrenics when they told the Emergency Room doctor that they were hearing voices or sounds.[19] Once on the ward, they allegedly acted perfectly normally, but the psychiatric staff continued to perceive their behaviour as evidence of psychopathology. Rosenhan claimed that this was evidence that set (or context) influences perceptions, and that the psychiatric staff overdiagnosed and, in a sense, created the mental illness by the mere act of diagnosing or labelling. Rosenhan's work has been soundly criticized for its lack of logic and honesty.[20] Far from decisively attacking the validity of diagnoses, his study merely demonstrates that a psychiatrist or psychiatric staff can be fooled when assuming that persons seeking help are truthful in their descriptions about themselves.

Critics of psychiatry also cite the certification and detention of dissidents in the USSR and their compulsory treatment by means of major tranquillizing drugs as testifying to the spurious nature not only of Russian but of all psychiatric diagnoses and to the essentially coercive and punitive nature of the treatments employed in psychiatric hospitals. It is rare for critics to refer to the fact that almost the entire psychiatric world, as also a number of intrepid Russian psychiatrists, have not merely condemned such practices,[21] but have been able to pinpoint specifically the vague, idiosyncratic and unvalidated character of the diagnostic criteria (e.g. 'sluggish schizophrenia') that have formed their starting point.

But if isolated examples of abuse are allowed to form the basis for sweeping generalizations, arguments can be conjured up to condemn not only psychiatry but every specialty within medicine. Not all surgical operations or medical treatments in current use are strictly necessary. This is not mentioned here in an attempt to condone Western psychiatric abuses, but to place such abuses within a broader medical and social context. No system designed and implemented by human beings is devoid of error or abuse. Yet, taken as a whole, the contributions of medical practice and medical science have been among the most constructive, humane and beneficient achievements of the human spirit.

The argument from the 'noble savage'

There are commonalities and differences between such leading critics of psychiatry as Basaglia, Foucault, Laing and Szasz. Basaglia is a Marxist; Foucault's politics veer towards the left, and Szasz's towards the right, although his attack on psychiatry is frequently used by Marxists who ignore the strong libertarian components of his philosophy. Laing remains, in essence, an apolitical mystic, although he appeared in his early writings to flirt with Marxism. Despite these differences, there is much common ground in their interpretations of the origins and character of mental illness, and in their disdain for the type of methodology and evidence which is expected of historians, scholars and scientists who wish to have their work taken seriously.

Much that they possess in common can be traced back to Rousseau, the intellectual godfather of Foucault and Laing and, in a special sense, of Szasz. Basaglia moves off in a more radical direction and will be considered in the next section. The idea of the 'noble savage' who 'heeding the stirrings of his heart rather than the weight of reason was kindly and pure' is found most clearly in Laing, and obliquely in Foucault. Rosseau portrayed an image of a utopian era in which man, if he could only follow the instincts given him by nature, would be innocent and happy; man is naturally and inherently good.

Civilization corrupts man in body and mind. Rousseau writes: 'In becoming social and enslaved, he becomes weak, timorous, and servile, and his soft, effeminate way of life completes the enervation of both his strength and his courage.'[22] According to Rousseau, man in a state of nature is healthy, and dies either of wounds or old age. It is civilization which causes disease, more rapidly than medicine can give us remedies. The causes of disease are as follows:

Extreme inequality in ways of living, with excessive idleness for some people and excessive work for others; the ease with which we can arouse and satisfy our appetites and our sensuality; the overrefined foods of the rich, which nourish them with warming juices and plague them with indigestion; the unwholesome food of the poor, who usually do not even have enough of it to satisfy their hunger, and therefore overload their stomachs whenever they have the opportunity; insufficient sleep; excesses of all kinds; immoderate outbursts of all the passions; fatigue; mental exhaustion; the countless sorrows and irritations that afflict people in all walks of life and constantly gnaw at the human soul – these are the pernicious proofs that most of our ills are of our own making, and that we could have avoided nearly all of them by keeping the simple, regular, and solitary way of life prescribed by nature. If nature meant man to be healthy, I might almost venture to say that the state of reflection is an unnatural state, and that a meditating man is a perverted animal.[23]

This image of an idyllic golden age, of man before the Fall, of the noble savage, has strong appeal to the Romantic within each of us, and partially provides an explanation for the indiscriminate idolization by contemporary youth of these themes in Laing and Foucault. 'Man is born free; and everywhere he is in chains. One thinks himself the master of others, and still remains a greater slave than they.'[24] Rousseau provides the moral condemnation and myth which are applied to the mid-twentieth century by Laing, Foucault and, in a somewhat different context, Ivan Illich.[25] Civilization destroys the noble savage: it inculcates fear, stifles creativity, exalts mediocrity and materialism, enforces conformity, and literally is the major cause of most of man's diseases.

Unlike Szasz, Laing and Foucault do not consistently refute the existence of mental illness. In some of their writings, the sufferings that are the essence of mental illness are advanced as evidence of the perniciousness of 'bourgeois' society. According to Laing, our social order creates mental illness; however, mental illness also serves as man's escape, from the personal alienation caused by society, back to the more primitive, instinctual, honest, uninhibited, and therefore morally superior style of life – that of the child and the savage, before the loss of innocence.

Rousseau (1762):

Before prejudices and human institutions have corrupted our natural inclinations, the happiness of children, like that of men, consists in the use of their freedom.[26]

Laing (1967):

As adults, we have forgotten most of our childhood, not only its contents but its flavour; as men of the world, we hardly know of the existence of the inner world: we barely remember our dreams, and make little sense of them when we do . . . Our capacity to think, except in the service of what we are dangerously deluded in supposing is our self-interest and in conformity with common sense, is pitifully limited.[27]

Rousseau, however, acknowledges that he speaks in allegory, and he cannot be expected to have had the medical knowledge presumed of Laing. Thus Rousseau may truly have believed that man in a state of nature does not suffer from diseases. He did not appreciate that natural man, living solitarily (a myth in itself) and away from civilization, is still prey to sleeping sickness (encephalitis) and malaria if he lives in a tropical climate; thyroid deficiency if he inhabits an area of insufficient iodides in the diet; malnutrition if there are droughts or famines; intestinal parasites if these are endemic; birth defects, diabetes or near-sightedness; depressions and schizophrenia if the genetic *and* other determinants of these illnesses are present. But we must assume that Laing is familiar with these facts.

To the myth of natural man, Foucault adds a Marxist colouring by postulating that the social oppression of the innocent person, whose destiny is to become a victim of mental illness, emanates from 'capitalist' society and, most specifically, from the 'bourgeois' family with its tyrannical father. Within this family, those who do not conform are made into scapegoats. The process of coercive conformity is continued by governmental and social institutions, churches, schools and, in adult life, marriage and the meretricious values that permeate 'bourgeois' society.

Psychiatrists, according to the antipsychiatry writers, are 'mind police' who form part of the 'bourgeois' power structure. Psychiatrists are alleged to have become willing instruments for the social control of those deviants whose 'radical voice' (Foucault) threatens the established order and its moral values. The deception perpetrated by psychiatry consists in its use of the respectable cloak of medicine to attach a disease label on those whose deviance threatens to undermine the power of the 'ruling classes'. This disease label serves to camouflage and invalidate the significance of the deviants' actions and to nullify their political effect. The social role of psychiatry is 'to obscure and indeed to deny the ethical dilemmas of life and to transform them into medical and technical problems susceptible to "professional solutions" '.[28] And the mental hospital, yet another tool for controlling subversion of society, has been created 'to promote certain values and performances and to suppress others'.[29]

There is a dark side, however, to Rousseau's doctrine of the noble savage which Laing and Foucault ignore, but which is picked up by Szasz. Szasz has little interest in the inherent goodness of man, and one finds no evidence that he might subscribe to such a notion. Unlike Laing, who commiserates with long-suffering humanity, Szasz appears to be an *Übermensch* élitist who, utilizing the umbrella of a libertarian philosophy, has scant sympathy for persons in poor health, especially those who are not able to care for themselves because they are marginally endowed with the basic biological features and skills needed for survival – common sense, intelligence, capacity for reciprocal emotional attachments, emotional stability, ability to work, absence of psychosis. His viewpoint is very reminiscent of a pre-Darwinian version of the theme of survival of the fittest found in Rousseau:

I would not take on a sickly and ill-constituted child, were he to live until eighty. I want no pupil always useless to himself and others, involved uniquely with preserving himself, whose body does damage to the education of the soul. What would I be doing in vainly lavishing my cares on him other than doubling society's loss and taking two men from it instead of one?[30]

Rousseau, in his later works, consistently attacks medicine, not so much on the basis of its demonstrated inefficacy and even dangerousness to the health of the patient, but more on ideological grounds. Medicine focuses man's attention on illness and ways of avoiding pain and death rather than on allowing nature to decide who shall survive and who shall die.

Szasz too holds that those afflicted with what are generally considered mental illnesses, such as suicidal depressions or schizophrenia, if they lack the sense, will or ability to obtain treatment, should be allowed to deteriorate or die. He sees nothing inequitable or incongruous in the healthy, righteous and strong in their health, telling the sick, who might not have asked for their diseases, deficiencies and incapacities, on just what special conditions treatment might be available.

Each of psychiatry's critics takes from Rousseau what is compatible with his viewpoint: Szasz the notion that special effort ought not to be expended in taking care of the sick, Foucault and Laing the romantic idea of a noble savage living in a golden age that never existed. In arguing from myth and allegory, they escape the requirement to offer evidence which might support their assertions; Laing, like Rousseau, can merely claim that something is true because his instinct, his heart, tell him so. Bertrand Russell has described the flaws in such a position in characteristic fashion:

Apart from the fictitious character of Rousseau's 'natural man', there are two objections to the practice of basing beliefs as to objective fact upon the emotions of the heart. One is that there is no reason whatever to suppose that such beliefs will be true; the other is, that the resulting beliefs will be private, since the heart says different things to different people. Some savages are persuaded by the 'natural light' that it is their duty to eat people, and even Voltaire's savages, who are led by the voice of reason to hold that one should only eat Jesuits, are not wholly satisfactory.[31]

The case appears somewhat different with Foucault and Szasz. Foucault provides evidence, and to some, the range of his arcane references has been overwhelming. However, repeated attempts by more conventional psychologists and historians to verify Foucault's 'evidence' have been unsuccessful.[32] Maher and Maher in the course of several years of investigation tried to discover the sources for Foucault's *stultifera navis* – the ships of fools that, according to Foucault, were used to transport (and thereby segregrate) the unwanted mentally ill from medieval city to city in an endless criss-crossing of the waterways of Europe.[33] Such dramatic imagery, symbolic of 'the great disquiet suddenly dawning on the horizon of European culture at the end of the Middle Ages', provides a critical piece of historical evidence in Foucault's tale. It has been canonized in official histories of psychology, along with several other misconceptions concerning the recognition and care of mental illness in the Middle Ages. In the Mahers' own words:

There is no evidence that any actual ships of fools put to sea with groups of the mentally ill in their indefinite custody. It seems probable that individual lunatics were sometimes transported away from towns into which they had wandered by a variety of means and that these occasionally included ships. There is some evidence that in the 14th and 15th centuries, as now, such burdensome persons were returned to the town or parish from whence they had come and which was responsible for their care.[34]

Szasz, unlike Foucault, offers no evidence. He is a rationalist, who proves by impeccable logic that mental illness is not illness. Nowhere does he offer a reasoned response to those who suggest that his logic is grounded on premises that are in disagreement with an impressive and growing body of evidence. Arguing from a self-contained logical system, and believing his premises and definitions to be self-evident, Szasz has little need of evidence. History, genetics, clinical and experimental data, and the data from objective evaluation of the assertions of labelling theorists clash with his premises and conclusions. But they can be ignored.

One must ask of Laing, Foucault, Szasz and others: How could their arguments be refuted? What sorts of evidence could be offered to cast doubt upon their theories, or to falsify them? The answer is that they are protected and rendered inviolate forever from any such challenge. The theories of Foucault, Laing, Szasz and their progeny can be used to explain all mental disease in all cultures and races at all times. It follows that they can explain nothing. They seek to prove a negative: that mental diseases as observed down the ages do not exist.

The argument of social control

Szasz and Laing, both practising psychiatrists and psychotherapists, agree that mental hospitals are prisons. According to Szasz, 'those who work in them are jailers and torturers'. One might well ask what Szasz and Laing offer as alternative proposals for those persons unable to endure their mental suffering and for whom a psychiatric diagnosis provides the initial step in attending to and alleviating their distress. One searches in vain for meaningful answers to such questions. Szasz seems to favour the provision of care by psychotherapists, but only if it occurs as a private contractual arrangement between a therapist and a self-designated patient. He also encourages those who seek his help 'to adopt a critical attitude towards all rules of conduct significant to him [the patient] and to maximize his free choice in adopting either socially accepted or unaccepted rules of conduct'.[35] This attitude presupposes that those who go to psychiatrists are calm, rational, functioning citizens who happen to have a few interpersonal problems that they wish to discuss with a trained psychotherapist. It is difficult to conceive how such advice could exert any influence whatsoever upon serious forms of mental illness and the many disruptions they cause in the lives of patients and their families.

One seeks in vain among Szasz's multitudinous pages for information regarding the results obtained by his approach. It would seem that those who suffer in mind will have to await the establishment of some more equitable social order before obtaining relief. The social and economic characteristics of such a utopian order remain shrouded in obscurity. Having regard to the finding of transcultural psychiatry that mental illness exists in all cultures, we would need more evidence than we are given before accepting the implicit prediction that citizens of some truly non-capitalist, non-bourgeois or libertarian society of the future would be free from schizophrenia, manic-depressive illness and other forms of mental suffering.

If we wish to appreciate, however, the results of putting Foucault's, Laing's and Szasz's theories into action on a large scale, we can look at the impact Basaglia has had on mental health care in Italy. It is interesting to juxtapose the writings of Basaglia and Szasz, since they disagree so fundamentally on which values and performances the mental patients threaten and the psychiatric establishment protects. But they both agree that persons are held in mental hospitals because they are seen as subversive to the social order. Whereas Foucault and Szasz have confined their activism to the world of words and ideas, Basaglia has actually been the architect of the most radical revision of mental health laws and the most extensive elimination of mental hospitals in the Western industrialized world. Basaglia was the medical director of the San Giovanni mental hospital in Trieste from 1971 to 1978 and presided over the partial dismantling of this hospital and the corresponding establishment of community facilities to care for the discharged patients. In 1974 he founded Psichiatria Democratica, a movement which appealed to trade unions, student activists, populists and, interestingly enough, the right wing legislators who saw in the closing of mental hospitals a way to reduce government expenditure. The movement became very popular and was responsible for the passage in 1978 of Law 180 which banned admission to mental hospitals of new patients and the re-admission of old patients. The law theoretically established 15-bed, short-term psychiatric units in general hospitals and made involuntary commitment so difficult (it required the signature of the mayor of the town) and so brief (48 hours, or renewed approval by the mayor and a judge) as to be virtually impossible.[36]

While Basaglia does not deny the existence of mental illness, his view of it is ideologically driven and very naive and, in a sense, very callous, despite the appearance of great concern. Basaglia views medicine in general as intimately linked to a capitalist society which defines the productive as 'well' and unproductive as 'sick'. He writes:

Medicine, entrusted with the treatment of everything that has been set within the sphere of illness, conceals the fundamental contradiction between the separation of the productive and the unproductive which then becomes opposition between 'sane' and 'sick' ... It is the appearance of the clinic which seems to indicate that the identification of 'unproductive' with 'sick' has been reached, as has the integration of medicine and productive organization. What production rejects is 'sick' and must subsequently be isolated and cared for by its institutions ... The contradiction re-emerges when deviation from the psychic norm (madness) falls, as sickness, within medicine's sphere or competence.[37]

Elsewhere, Basaglia states:

'Mental illness' as we know it was seen not as what the mental hospital cures, but as what it creates: from this source emanate both the categories of disorder and the fundamental meaning of mental illness as something to be segregated and contained.[38]

Thus Basaglia had two motivations for working toward the abolition of mental hospitals. The first stemmed from his belief that the hospital was the critical link in causing and perpetuating mental illness, and that only when there would be no mental hospital for society to confine its unproductive members in could there be a solid effort to protect, cure and rehabilitate those persons made 'mentally ill' by the class structure itself. The second motivation, however, saw the mental patients as the vanguard of the revolution. It callously ejected them from hospitals so they would be more conspicuous in the streets and serve as living examples of the contradictions inherent in capitalist societies. In Basaglia's words:

The project [creating a new awareness of the social oppression implicit in mental illness] was therefore more akin to the political struggles which broke out in other areas of social life during the 1960s, breaking up established institutions and exposing their shortcomings, than to avant-garde psychiatric experiments like the 'therapeutic community' in England, or 'la psychiatrie institutionelle' in France.[39]

The hardships and havoc wrought by Law 180 were not long in coming.

Whatever the shortcomings of the mental hospitals in Italy prior to 1978, there was some supervision and accountability, and patients were at least fed and clothed. Basaglia, and the legislators, acted as though schizophrenia, manic-depressive illnesses, epileptic psychoses and toxic conditions were all uniformly caused by inequities of power and wealth in society. It was as though brain and body and individual life experiences (such as early death of a parent) did not exist. Several articles have been published recently documenting the disaster that occurred in Italy. Jones and Poletti travelled through Italy (from the Swiss border to the extreme south) in April 1984 and visited many mental health centres.[40] Their observations have been verified by Papeschi[41] and Sarteschi, Cassano, Mauri and Petracca.[42] The institutions are still standing and in use, except that they are deteriorating because few funds are available for their repair and maintenance. Patients are still present, although in lesser numbers, and are now called 'guests'. Some hospital buildings have been renamed nursing homes and their patients are now called 'geriatric patients'. Few staff are present and no programmes. Similarly, in the absence of a national initiative or funding, local regions have done little to commit resources or develop community programmes. The prisons hold more mental patients than formerly; the number of homeless mentally ill persons wandering the cities is also greatly increased.

Jones and Poletti describe their observations as follows:

We looked for the pleasant, informal Psycho-Social Centres and were able to visit only one – a homely Italian version of an English day centre, run by an occupational therapist. Most were in fact no more than out-patient clinics, with some community nurses (untrained, but with mental hospital experience) attached. As we went south, the provision became less, and the the problems greater. In Salerno, there were only 50 Diagnosis and Cure beds for a population of one million, and no other services of any kind . . .

Private nursing homes were springing up on all sides, and there was no form of public inspection, though public funds (from the USSLs) were being used to support patients in many. One psychiatrist described the private homes in his own area as 'basically horrible'. Having visited one, we saw no reason to dispute his verdict – though there may be better provision in other areas, the potentialities for abuse of the system are considerable.[43]

The experience in Italy dwarfs the failures of deinstitutionalization in the United States. If one wanted to know what would happen if Foucault's or Szasz's theories were put into practice, one could look to the events in Italy for instruction.[44] The exploitation of mental patients as pawns in an ideological struggle ignores the realities of their disabilities and legitimate needs for responsible, supervised and accountable medical care. There are several Bills being prepared for the repeal of Law 180 by the Italian legislature.

Steps towards solutions

We are guided by two basic principles which underlie all of our discussion. The first, already introduced, is that issues of human behaviour and human responsibility are complex, and that it can only be misleading to pretend otherwise. The second principle, in itself a refinement or derivative of these epistemological complexities, is that there are no sharp divisions found in nature, although for pragmatic purposes we have to act as though there are. Even the events of birth and death, those two seemingly unambiguous beginning and end points of life which, if nothing else were certain, could at least be counted on to provide us with clear anchors of stable judgement, are themselves now thrown open to question. It matters little that the impetus for debate is moral-political in the case of the beginning of life, and moral-legalistic in the case of the termination of life. The debates have merely emphasized that, even here, there are no generally accepted absolute limits. Indeed once the position is accepted that life begins before birth, we lose our only precise and unarguable boundary-line. Similarly, once we acknowledge that life can extend beyond the cessation of a heartbeat, then the actual moment of death is decided by the vagaries of a technological rather than a vital organic process. If there is no agreement as to when life begins and ends, how much greater is our uncertainty in deciding where health ends and illness begins? This question has innumerable subdivisions: Where does normal blood pressure end and hypertension begin? does cognitive impairment in old age end and dementia begin? Where does idiosyncratic thinking end and delusional and autistic thinking begin? Where does sadness end and melancholia begin?

Despite these uncertainties, the practical daily necessities of clinical medicine require that illnesses be defined, identified and treated without falling into philosophical paralysis. This necessity establishes what is perhaps the most fundamental dilemma in medicine: how to cluster similar conditions into patterns of syndromes and diseases with a minimum of overlap and a maximum of systematic import. By systematic import we refer to the power that a concept has in providing additional information (explanation, prediction and understanding) which was not known prior to the introduction of that particular concept.[45] For example, based upon our observations of the regularity with which feelings of sadness and hopelessness are accompanied by attitudes of self-blame, sleep disturbances, decreased appetite and sexual interest, and impaired concentration, we develop the hypothesis that this whole collection of signs and symptoms forms a group of related entities which we call depression. When we have identified individuals who exhibit such behaviours, we can proceed to investigate their family, and in this manner postulate several probable patterns of genetic transmission of mood disorders, including a greater than expected prevalence of relatives with problems of alcohol abuse. We can also obtain additional information about depressed patients as a class: that their overall mortality rate as well as their suicide rate is higher than in the general population, and that recognizable subgroups within the larger class of disorders called depression respond differently to different treatments, at times with total remission of the illness.

Our ability to describe a syndrome called depression and to identify individuals who have this condition, and our subsequent ability to discover additional features (suicide, affected relatives) does not cause us to forget that depression is an ordinary aspect of human and animal life, that all persons have variations of mood and degrees of depression at times, and that it is often difficult to distinguish those depressions that seem to arise from unfortunate circumstances (grief, loss) from those that seem to arise in the absence of external precipitating factors.

The values of classification

These difficulties reflect an inevitable tension in all scientific endeavours. There is heuristic value in classifying seemingly continuous functions into separate categories; there is an equally compelling value in not inventing differences which as far as we can tell do not exist. For most scientific fields, including medicine, the practical gains of a classification system that assigns individuals to particular categories far outweigh whatever information is lost in such an activity. Thus, as we have indicated, there is great practical advantage, especially in terms of treatment, in being able to recognize that an individual with certain specific characteristics of sadness, insomnia and suicidal ruminations satisfies the defining criteria of a category called depressive illness.

The risk of such a classification system, however, is that it tends to reify the categories, as though depression or pneumonia were things which exist apart from the person with the illness. In addition, the separation of diseases into distinct categories tends to obscure the relatedness of diseases to each other, and to focus on single causes at the expense of an appreciation of the multiple levels of causation in the development of illness. This is most obvious in the artificial distinctions between mental and physical illnesses which Szasz and others exploit in their arguments.

Mental versus physical disease: a false dichotomy

To be precise, even the term 'mental illness' is a misnomer; it is based upon an outdated distinction between body and mind that remains a philosophical, but not a biological, dilemma. All illnesses eventually interfere with functioning in psychological, social, economic and physical spheres, place the affected person at a biological disadvantage, bring suffering to self and others, are present at times without the ill person recognizing it, have acute and chronic forms, and are associated with increased mortality. 'Physical' and 'mental' factors can bring on or exacerbate illnesses: stress can lead to peptic ulcers and hypertension; exhaustion, malnutrition and endocrine disorders can lead to emotional disorders. In fact, all metabolic, infectious and organic diseases will affect cognition, mood and behaviour if the delicate homeostatic functions (blood pH, serum electrolyte levels, red blood cell oxygen carrying capacity) which influence them are altered significantly.

Most importantly, the differentiation of complex conditions into purely physical or purely mental illnesses, or even the attachment of appropriate weights to the biological, psychological and social aspects of illness in different types of cases, is frequently very difficult or impossible. For example, in a post-partum psychosis – which is severe and life-threatening to the mother as well as disruptive with serious long-term implications for the development of bonding and the future relationship between mother and child – how is one to distinguish the contribution of the hormonal and metabolic changes attendant upon pregnancy and delivery from the psychological and symbolic impact of becoming a mother? It is pure sophistry to attempt such a division; mind and body cannot be separated.

An examination of persons suffering from depression provides the best illustration of the inseparability of physical and emotional components in the development of illness. Depressive illness arises from the interaction of many factors: hereditary predisposition to depression expressed possibly through effects on central nervous regulation of mood stability; hormonal factors and alterations in diurnal rhythm; the availability of correct proportions of the chemical transmitters which carry impulses across the neuronal synapse; a range of biochemical factors which affect sensitivity and responsiveness of receptor sites at the nerve endings; general physical health; state of nutrition; fatigue, and the presence of concomitant illness; life events such as loss of a parent in childhood; situational factors such as marital relationships, family dynamics and employment situation; values and attitudes that arise from spiritual and religious beliefs; and personal factors such as self-esteem and sense of control over one's destiny. These are factors that combine, in unfavourable cases, to bring about depression in the individual. It would perhaps be more accurate to state that the depression is comprised of these factors. We can then say that the person is depressed or has a depression. The illness does not reside in a single organ or system. There are profound changes in the brain and cerebrospinal fluid, in the molecular composition of submicroscopic structures, in the hypothalamic-pituitary-adrenal axis and other endocrine systems,[46] in resistance to infection and malignant tumours,[47] in the dynamics of the circulatory system, in platelet function[48] and, of course, in the conscious awareness of saddened mood, lack of energy and initiative, and lowered morale. There are also profound changes in the depressed person's social network, with impact on spouse, children, relatives and friends. The following case illustrates some of these points.

> A 52-year-old, married assembly-line worker with a good work record despite intermittent alcohol problems and marital jealousy sustains a penetrating knee injury at work. The knee joint becomes infected, necessitating surgery. Following surgery the patient appears to do well for a week, but while working on a leg-exercise device in the hospital to strengthen the knee, he develops a rash and then an infection where the exercise machine rubs against his skin.

Over the next three years the patient is hospitalized six times for severe skin infections and a reinfected knee, necessitating two more surgical procedures. The skin lesions, full of pus and smelling foully, seem to clear up in the hospital, only to recur fulminantly when the patient returns home. The patient begins to appear both depressed and angry. He sleeps poorly and loses interest in his family. He spends six to twelve hours at a time in the bathroom, washing his sores, picking off the scabs with tweezers and razors, scraping his skin until it bleeds at many points. He applies ointment to his skin, rebandages his arms, legs and abdomen, but then starts the entire process over again. He refuses to leave the house, stating that he smells too badly. He is belligerent to his family when they try to interrupt his procedures. His occupation of the only bathroom forces his family to use the neighbour's bathroom. His prolonged use of leg bandages lead to atrophy of his muscles and mild contractures of his knee joints, such that he is confined to a wheelchair and can barely support his weight when standing. He despairs of ever going to work and makes oblique references to shooting himself with a gun from his gun collection.

During one period of hospitalization, when his doctor remarks that his skin infections never affect his back or other areas he cannot reach and that he must be spreading the infection, the patient becomes furious, discharges himself from hospital, and refuses to approach another hospital for a year. However, the skin infection continues unabated and the patient's morale and relationship with family further deteriorate. He can think and speak only of his skin infections. Such is his condition when his family insists that he return to hospital.

What can be said of such a person that would do full justice to his complex medical and psychological problems? That all of this might be an understandable series of responses to an industrial accident or that none of this would have happened if not for the initial accident? But there are many similar accidents with relatively uneventful recoveries. That the man is depressed and that his increasing disinterest in his family, his irritability, and morbid preoccupation with his skin infections are manifestations of this depression? That his basic personality structure was paranoid (there is inconclusive evidence for this) which decompensated under the stress of the illness? That his daily twelve-hour episodes of ritualistic self-mutilation represent a delusional state, in which the patient is convinced that he is lethally contaminated with some unclean substance and requires almost constant decontamination? That he is intentionally and self-consciously inflicting damage on himself either because of neurotic masochistic needs or to maintain the secondary gains which his invalid status provides?

Realism and humility are required for any reasonable response. We do not know what has happened and probably never will, for there are no simple answers or formulae, nor can we read his mind. Even though he may improve, perhaps recover, we will never have more than an incomplete understanding of what has happened to this man, much less be able to disentangle the psychological from the medical components. It is intellectually and technically impossible to provide a complete description of his 'medical' disease – the skin infections – without including in such a description the bizarre behaviours of his 'mental' disease – the elaborate rituals of attacking his scabs with tweezers and razor which spread the infection and prevented healing. And it is equally impossible to encompass his 'mental' disease – his behaviours and whatever internal psychological processes may have been occurring – without also including in such a description a complete account of his skin infections and initial knee injury.

But of course none of this occurs in a vacuum. This man has a nervous system and a personality built up of all that has happened to him and all that he has done, together with all that his genetic and physical-somatic constitution bring. Thus somewhere in the description of either the patient or his disease must be included the piece of information that, when he was 10 years old, his alcoholic father committed suicide. Also included must be a description of his relationship with his wife and children, the manner in which it evolved over the years, and how it interacted with his illness. At some point in our investigation, or our attempt at understanding, we come upon the practical necessity of arriving at clear and constructive decisions about what we are to do for him. This compels us to offer the best tentative diagnoses and the most relevant treatment programmes we can devise.

Part of our success in modern science has been made possible by our practice of separating out for investigation and experimentation discrete pieces of larger problems. In providing care for this man, we will treat his skin infections with antibiotics, his mood and thought disturbances with antidepressant and/or antipsychotic medication, his damaged and incapacitated knee with rehabilitation therapies, his profound demoralization with psychotherapy, his deteriorating marital relationship with family counselling, and his extended unemployment with vocational guidance. But such compartmentalized treatment, established pragmatically in this age of technical and efficient subspecialization, does not justify a concept of a compartmentalized man. We need not lose sight of him as a unique and special person.

The essence of the case presented by the antipsychiatry writers can be succinctly expressed; it is a restatement of what has come to be known as the traditional medical model, in a new guise. It advances a view that only those forms of human suffering which can be shown unequivocally to be caused by biological factors in the sense of structural lesions or specific metabolic alterations can be regarded as diseases. All other forms of suffering of body and mind, unaccompanied by such lesions, are not to be considered diseases or illnesses.

In truth, such considerations of what constitutes disease may pose social, moral or ethical problems but not medical ones. In this book we will argue that adherence to a 'lesion-based' medical model is to apply the technique of Procrustes to all of medicine, including psychiatry. It is to limit the scope of every discipline within medicine in a manner that is likely to augment rather than mitigate the disability or distress of those who suffer.

The central arguments of antipsychiatry are simplistic. They ignore the obdurate and complex nature of problems involving mental and physical disease. The absence of clean lines of demarcation between mental and bodily disorders as shown by a convincing body of factual evidence is ignored. The ancient and unsolved problems of mind–body interaction are resolved at a single stroke by a Solomon-like judgement which sharply separates mind from body. The antipsychiatry writers establish a spurious dichotomy, with mind and body having little to do with each other.

We will examine here whether the partition of the practice of medicine into conditions of biological causation on the one hand and problems concerning the quality of life on the other is supported by clinical observation and objective enquiry.

2 Disorders of the mind and the role of medicine in historical perspective

In their concern for a convincing argument, the antipsychiatry writers distort the historical record to make it fit their theories. Their polemics often display ignorance of the history of mental disorders, the historical context in which past events occurred, and the subject matter of psychiatry itself. Reporting history correctly and accurately would weaken their arguments considerably and contradict certain myths about the past which have great popular appeal.

These myths, although advanced by different writers from different points of view, are interrelated. First, there is the myth that the profession of medicine did not concern itself with disorders of the mind until the eighteenth and nineteenth centuries when it became clear that such an interest would bring power and money to physicians. Thus, Foucault writes that the medical takeover of the asylum came about at the end of the eighteenth century, after the release from confinement of vagabonds, paupers, debtors and libertines. Only the mad remained. This brought about a new relation between insanity and medical thought; 'mental disease, with the meanings we now give it, is made possible'.[1] Similarly, Scull alleges that it was in the early 1800s that the medical profession first began to take an interest in lunacy.[2]

The second myth is that medicine's takeover of mental disorders resulted in Draconian measures of institutionalization and oppressive treatments. Before this there had been a golden period in which the carefree schizophrenic, melancholic, demented and delirious patients (before they are labelled as such) roamed the countryside under the benevolent protection of family, church and society. According to the myth there were several reasons why this was so, the major one being that medicine had not yet acquired the power to exercise control over the insane and physicians were not yet labelling them in this manner. According to Scull, it was contact with society's official experts (in this case, the physicians), rather than manifestations of specific behavioural or mental disturbances, which most firmly and legitimately designated these people as madmen in the eyes of laymen. In other words, when a member of the family sat mutely and stared at the walls for several days, or talked incoherently, or ran naked out of the house, the family was unable to appreciate that the person was ill until a physician pronounced him so. No evidence is ever offered for this assertion, which flies in the face of common sense and experience.[3] Rather, as Kathleen Jones has pointed out, Scull's arguments consist mainly of 'trendy, in-group terminology' which serves to strike a political pose and win the approval of sympathetic groups.[4] The terms, dramatic and somewhat inflammatory, have to carry the weight of the argument in the absence of evidence and reasonable alternatives. Thus Scull and other radical sociologists speak of 'decarceration', 'social control', 'deinstitutionalisation' and 'advanced capitalist societies' when referring to governmental efforts to establish community care of chronic mental illnesses. Jones proceeds by allowing Scull's invective to speak for itself. First it was 'incarceration' against which he argued; now 'decarceration' is the object of the same attack, with an unacknowledged acceptance of the fact that there really *are* some people who are so disturbed that they do require care and protection in an institution.

Laing goes straight to the heart of the romantic perspective of mental illness, which he views as the only reasonable response of a sensitive soul to the insanity of the daily world:

what we call 'normal' is a product of repression, denial, splitting, projection, introjection and other forms of destructive action on experience ... There are forms of alienation that are relatively strange to statistically 'normal' forms of alienation. The 'normally' alienated person, by reason of the fact that he acts more or less like everyone else, is taken to be sane. Other forms of alienation that are out of step with the prevailing state of alienation are those that are labelled by the 'normal' majority as bad or mad. The condition of alienation, of being asleep, of being unconscious, of being out of one's mind, is the condition of the normal man.[5]

Laing blames our 'bourgeois' society both for causing schizophrenia and then for treating the condition so callously. Our society is insane; the schizophrenic recognizes this and flees in an attempt to find sanity through madness. Laing writes:

Perhaps we will come to accord to so-called schizophrenics who have come back to us, perhaps after years, no less respect than the often no less lost explorers of the Renaissance. If the human race survives, future men will, I suspect, look back on our enlightened epoch as a veritable Age of Darkness ... They will see that what we call 'schizophrenia' was one of the forms in which, often through quite ordinary people, the light began to break through the cracks in our all-too-closed minds.[6]

Susan Sontag takes issue with the romantic veneer thus painted over some of the most life-impoverishing diseases of mankind. In her book *Illness as Metaphor* she writes of the one-time view of tuberculosis:

If it is still difficult to imagine how the reality of such a dreadful disease could be transformed so preposterously, it may help to consider our own era's comparable act of distortion, under the pressure of the need to express romantic attitudes about the self. The object of distortion is not, of course, cancer – a disease which nobody has managed to glamorize (though it fulfills some of the functions as a metaphor that TB did in the nineteenth century). In the twentieth century, the repellent harrowing disease that is made the index of a superior sensitivity, the vehicle of 'spiritual' feelings and 'critical' discontent, is insanity ... In the twentieth century the cluster of metaphors and attitudes formerly attached to TB are split up and are parceled out to two diseases. Some features of TB go to insanity: the notion of the sufferer as a hectic, reckless creature of passionate extremes, someone too sensitive to bear the horrors of the vulgar, everyday world. Other features of TB go to cancer – the agonies that can't be romanticized. Not TB but insanity is the current vehicle of our secular myth of self-transcendence. The romantic view is that illness exacerbates consciousness. Once that illness was TB; now it is insanity that is thought to bring consciousness to a state of paroxysmic enlightenment. The romanticizing of madness reflects in the most vehement way the contemporary prestige of irrational or rude (spontaneous) behaviour (acting-out), of that very passionateness whose repression was once imagined to cause TB, and is now thought to cause cancer.[7]

The implications of the labelling theorists' and Laing's romantic portrait of insanity are that there was less insanity in earlier times because no organization had been created for the purpose of labelling social deviants as insane. The myth continues that before the profession of medicine had officially been given the task of diagnosing and treating the insane, mental illness was not considered to be a medical condition and the mentally ill were treated with benign neglect. It is a contradiction of this thesis and a misreading of the historical record when the Middle Ages are also singled out to demonstrate the cruel and merciless manner in which society persecutes those who deviate from its norms. Although a Renaissance rather than a medieval phenomenon, there was little of benevolence in the bizarre confessions extracted during the trials of persons accused of witchcraft, often manifestly insane women whose self-accusations were liable to exceed the charges laid against them.

A third myth, principally associated with the labelling theorists, is that 'mental disorders' themselves, or rather 'primary deviance', comprise a number of benign and harmless variants of normal conduct such as rule breaking, legitimate dissent and idiosyncracy. This assumption ignores the intense misery and hardship created by schizophrenic or manic-depressive illness within families. It also turns a blind eye to the historical reality that, until quite recently, the majority of those diagnosed as mentally ill and admitted to mental hospitals suffered from organic conditions including epilepsy, severe mental retardation, dementia, delirious states, metabolic and toxic conditions, infectious illnesses and nutritional disorders. These conditions constituted a large proportion of the disorders seen and written about by physicians and laymen prior to the twentieth century.

In fact, medicine has always been involved with the care of the mentally ill; the accepted explanation of the cause of mental illness in Western civilization has historically been physiological rather than psychological or supernatural; and the labelling theorists have produced no evidence whatsoever to support their theories that the occurrence and symptomatology of the major mental illnesses are at all derived from a new social recognition and stigmatization.

There is an instructive passage in the Old Testament in I Samuel 21:10–16. The young David, fleeing the murderous jealousy and rage of King Saul, takes refuge with his enemy, Achish the king of Gath of the Philistine nation. However, David, wearing the sword of Goliath with which he beheaded the Philistine giant, is recognized by the servants of the king. When they comment about Saul slaying his thousands and David his ten thousands, David fears for his life:

And he changed his behaviour before them, and feigned himself mad in their hands, and scrabbled on the doors of the gate, and let his spittle fall down upon his beard. Then said Achish unto his servants, Lo, ye see the man is mad: wherefore then have ye brought him to me? Have I need of mad men, that ye have brought this fellow to play the mad man in my presence? Shall the fellow come into my house?[8]

It is clear from this passage that mental illness was a well-recognized condition in the Near East in 1000 BC, or certainly by 500 BC when the Scriptures were committed to writing. David would not otherwise have known how to feign madness nor could the Philistines have recognized it. We also are given a brief description of 'mad' behaviour: banging on the door and drooling down one's beard. Furthermore, we are told that an 'enlightened' attitude existed about mental illness, since David, in his desperation, had reasonable confidence that the Philistines would not harm a 'madman', even if an enemy. Although earlier passages refer to Saul's rages and terrors as caused by an evil spirit, no explanation is offered by the Philistines for David's alleged madness. The text is noteworthy for its absence of a demonic explanation.

Mental illness in antiquity

The Greeks developed two parallel theories of explanation and methods of treatment of mental illness, both of which are extant today. These theories are not mutually incompatible, and often seem to complement each other. The first is that of supernatural causation, the details of which may vary from culture to culture. The primary theme is that a spirit or demon inhabits the 'mad' person or causes the madness without actual possession. Alternatively God or one of many gods causes the madness, or a witch or sorcerer has cast a spell to cause the madness. The insanity may be seen as punishment, but this is not invariable; it may be a prank of an evil spirit, or a demonstration of God's power to cure insanity by driving out evil spirits, or a method of testing and purifying a soul.

Contemporaneously with this supernatural theory there developed a well-elaborated biological or medical theory of insanity. Although ignored by the antipsychiatry writers, this medical tradition has been unbroken since the time of Hippocrates (circa 400 BC). The dominant theme in the medical tradition for 2000 years has been the humoral theory, as clear a biological theory as one can find.[9] This theory perceives *all* illnesses, including mental illness, as stemming from imbalances in the natural humours (fluids) of the body. The theory of humours, which was well-developed and complex, included an elaborate regimen of treatments based upon the alleged qualities (hot, cold, dry, moist) of natural substances which would counteract the humoral imbalances. The adjunctive uses by the Romans of astrology and 'magical' stones and jewels were also considered rational, not superstitious. It was accepted as obvious that the planets, stars and the moon influence the human condition, including health and disease, and that certain stones and gems have inherent powers to cure. The latter notion was no more strange than our acceptance of the power of a magnet to attract iron by virtue of its magnetic qualities. In the light of the level of scientific knowledge at that time, the Romans' belief in the efficacy of planetary influence was no more fantastic than our belief in the existence of atoms which we cannot see or our casual explanation that objects fall to earth because of the 'force of gravity'.

Mental illness in the Middle Ages

The physiological tradition in medicine exemplified by the humoral theory was continuous from Hippocrates through Galen and Soranus to the writers of the later Roman empire and on into the Middle Ages. The Middle Ages provides an interesting illustration of the ideological misuse of history, first because it is the favourite theme of enlightened modernists who wish to show how far we have evolved from our barbarous past, and second because the antipsychiatry writers claim that the involvement of medicine with mental illness did not come about until the eighteenth century. This they can do only by ignoring the entire thousand-year period (AD 500–1500) of the Middle Ages. The proponents of this view would have us believe that all madness was considered to be supernaturally caused and that madmen were persecuted as witches and heretics. The historical record tells a different story.[10]

A distinction must be made, as in all ages, between the views of physicians and medical writers and those held by the general populace. This is especially important for the Middle Ages. To generalize from the demonological views which then gained a certain currency and to ignore the contribution of medical writers who were in a direct line of continuity with present medical science and scholarship is unbalanced and inaccurate. There were both lay and clerical practising physicians in the Middle Ages. There were also scholars who compiled Greek, Latin and, later, Arabic medical texts into encyclopaedic works, adding their own opinions, revising and at times plagiarizing freely. These works, without exception, were biological in description and aetiology.[11] The texts were organized according to topographical anatomy with mental illnesses being included in the section devoted to the head, and with no distinction being made between mental illness and other types of illness.

For example, in Isidore of Seville's (AD 560–636) *Etymologiae*,[12] in which a section (Book XI) is devoted to medicine, the account on chronic diseases begins with headache and proceeds to dimness of vision and vertigo attributed to inflation of the air-passages and blood vessels at the top of the head and resolution of the moisture there (Section 7). It continues with epilepsy (which is said to arise whenever the black bile develops in excess and is turned in its course to the brain) and proceeds to mania, melancholia, intermittent fevers, rheums, catarrhus or coryza (running nose), hoarseness, laryngitis, pneumonia, and so fourth. When discussing the medical causes of epilepsy Isidore even mentions that the common people call its sufferers 'lunatics' because of the influence of the moon's cycles.

Isidore was a prominent churchman who, as bishop of Seville, exemplified the religious belief, piety and dedication of an early seventh-century ecclesiastic. He believed in angels and demons, and would not dispute that these beings could cause disease or that the origin of sickness was sometimes to be found in sin. It was not incompatible for Isidore or other churchmen to believe both that disease was sent by God to punish or cleanse, and that imbalance of the humours accurately accounted for the underlying disease process. Such themes and others that followed are perhaps best illustrated by the recurrent epidemics of plague (Black Death) in the late Middle Ages, which were conceived both as vengeful acts of God and as physical diseases. Isidore was not a physician, and his writings on medicine, which were unimaginative and obdurate, were of little practical value. But they were highly influential in laying logical conceptual foundation for future medical texts.

During the early Middle Ages (AD 600–1000), while Europe was undergoing devastating and concurrent invasions by the Magyars, Norsemen and Saracens, most medical learning and knowledge, except that practised by lay physicians in Italy and in some of the more powerful ducal courts, was preserved within the monasteries. It is incorrect to say that the church suppressed medical learning and practice. It understandably stressed the primacy of spiritual over physical values, but the establishment of medical facilities in each monastery for the care of sick brethren was strongly encouraged.[13] The mistaken allegation that the church was anti-medical rests with the compelling need of certain writers to demonstrate that everything about the Middle Ages and the church was reprehensible. These writers include hostility to the practice of medicine among the church's crimes, but such an allegation has little substance. Its flimsy foundations are perhaps to be found in the fact that after AD 1000 the monasteries discouraged, or forbade, their members from practising medicine outside the monastery.[14] But this had much to do with the doctrinal disputes over whether monks should ever leave their monasteries for any reason and almost nothing to do with the actual practice of medicine.

With the flowering of the Middle Ages in the eleventh and twelfth centuries, the teaching and practice of medicine moved out of the monasteries and into cathedral schools, such as Chartres and Rheims, and the famous lay schools at Salerno and Montpellier.[15] Under both types of organization the medical writings and teachings remained biologically oriented and free from demonological speculations.

It might, however, be thought that, although medical texts and teaching showed little interest in sin and demons, the actual practice of medicine, and the beliefs of ordinary people in the Middle Ages, were infused with notions of punishment and demonological influences. There can be no question but that a two-tiered universe (natural and spiritual) was the dominant world-view at this time, and that all natural phenomena, including birth, death, accidents, diseases, good fortune, unseasonable weather, finding one's way home after being lost, unusual animal or insect behaviour, could be attributed to the influences of the supernatural world. Again, it must be emphasized that to the medieval mentality, natural and supernatural events were neither sharply differentiated nor incompatible, but much a part of the total world order. When God brought the ten plagues upon the Egyptians, they were natural plagues, not ghostly visitations. In any case, thinking one's afflictions to be a punishment for transgression is a human reaction common to all cultures.

The erroneous connection between sin and illness

Laing and Foucault and other antipsychiatry writers base their argument that medicine was not in the past involved with insanity in part on their assertion that in the Middle Ages insanity was uniformly attributed to sin, not illness. A detailed scrutiny of passing commentaries about illnesses from diverse *non-medical* medieval sources does not support the customary assumptions about medieval beliefs in the causal relationships between sin and illness and, especially, sin and insanity. This is the more remarkable considering that the authors of these pre-Crusade medieval chronicles and saints' lives were all clerics. The evidence is as follows: of fifty-seven references to insanity and possession in eleven pre-Crusade sources, only nine (16%) make reference to sin; of 396 references to illnesses in twenty-nine pre-Crusade sources, seventy-four (19%) make reference to sin.[16] Furthermore, in almost every case in which an illness was linked to sin, the medieval authors appeared to use this attribution for its propaganda value against an enemy of their patron saints, the monastery lands, or their religious values. There was no attribution of sin when, as in the overwhelming majority of descriptions of illnesses, a pious person became ill. There is an illustration of this latter point in Bede's *Life of Cuthbert* (seventh century), in which it is mentioned that the wife of the sheriff, *a good woman*, was possessed of a devil.[17] The woman threw herself about and was considered mad; she was cured by St Cuthbert at the request of her husband. Not only was any reference to sin omitted, but the text specifically mentions that she was a good woman. An example of a reference to insanity linked to sin is in Bede's *History of the English Church and People*, in which King Eadbald rejected Christianity and was subject to insanity.[18]

Additional evidence refuting the traditional position that early European psychiatric thought was dominated by demonology has been presented by

Neugebauer who, in a series of studies of medieval and early modern English incompetency hearings, demonstrated that 'The English government conducted mental status examinations of psychiatrically disabled individuals, using commonsense, naturalistic criteria of impairment.' Neugebauer further showed that 'etiological theories entertained by royal officials and laymen relied on physiological and psychological notions of psychiatric illness'. Causes of psychiatric problems included illness with fever, a blow received on the head, and a fear of one's father.[19]

Mental illness in the Renaissance

As the Middle Ages drew to a close, there was an increase both in demonological preoccupation and in scientific discovery. The major inquisitions, witch-hunts and witchburnings occurred in the Renaissance and pre-Enlightenment periods, not the Middle Ages.[20] But so did the discoveries of Galileo, Copernicus and Newton. There was a growth in secular medicine and a loosening of the ties between natural disease and supernatural underpinnings, so much so that by the seventeenth and eighteenth centuries philosophers and physicians alike could characterize the living person as a machine.

In passing it is interesting to comment that Descartes, whose mind–body dichotomy helped establish the notion of man as machine and still provides the rationale for the argument that mental illnesses are not really illnesses, had no difficulty himself in recognizing without qualifications the presence of madness. In his *Meditations on First Philosophy*, which established this dichotomy, Descartes thinks about the things which may be brought within the sphere of the doubtful.[21] He states that he cannot doubt that he

is here, seated by the fire, attired in dressing gown ... And how could I deny that these hands and this body are mine, were it not perhaps that I compare myself to certain persons, devoid of sense, whose cerebella are so troubled and clouded by the violent vapors of black bile, that they constantly assure us that they think they are kings when they are really quite poor, or that they are clothed in purple when they are really without covering, or who imagine that they have an earthenware head or are nothing but pumpkins or are made of glass. But they are mad, and I should not be any the less insane were I to follow examples so extravagant.

We can summarize this review of the evolution of concepts of disease including mental disease during the Middle Ages as follows. The theory and practice of medicine represented a fusion of Greek, Roman and Arabic physiological theories, Christian belief, and local pagan traditions. Mental illnesses were not considered different in nature from physical illnesses and were not singled out for special demonological preoccupation. In fact, all events were interpreted in terms of a dual universe and, in the broader sense, neither physical illnesses nor mental illnesses were treated differently from any other class of events. Life was harsh:

infant mortality was around 40%, life expectancy close to 30 years of age, famines and malnutrition were frequent, warfare was endemic, and medical treatment largely ineffective.[22] This was the background to the Middle Ages, and to extract from all this grimness the assertion that the mentally ill were treated especially badly or especially well is at variance with historical fact.

This latter point raises a further misconception of the antipsychiatry writers that prior to the great confinement of the indigent, criminals and mentally ill in the period 1650–1700 there was a golden age in the care of the insane. This is quite untrue. It is clear from descriptions of the insane in the Middle Ages and Renaissance that they were miserable individuals, wandering around in village and forest, taken from shrine to shrine, and sometimes tied up when they became too violent. They met with the full range of responses, from Christian support, through tolerance to persecution. They were treated with medical and natural remedies as well as saints' relics and pagan rituals. Throughout these centuries, medical theory and practice were as concerned with the mentally ill as with other medically ill persons. The consistent and fair treatment of the mentally ill was the result of the church's emphasis on Christian charity as well as medicine's emphasis on physiological causation. The eruption of demonological concerns and witchcraft trials in the sixteenth and seventeenth centuries reflects a disruption of the entire social fabric and was in no way an assault focused on the mentally ill. That the mentally ill were included is no matter for surprise. But it may have owed more to the lack of power and authority of those engaged in the practice of medicine than to any selective cruelty and harshness meted out to those with mental disorder.

3 The evidence from transcultural enquiries

It is one of the cornerstones of the critique advanced by antipsychiatrists that the concept and actual care of mental illness was not included within a broader concept of medical illness until the eighteenth and nineteenth centuries, when it profited the medical profession to do so. We have seen that this assertion is devoid of substance. Another constituent argument of this critique, intertwined with the first because both partake of the same logic, is the claim that there is no such thing as mental illness. It is asserted that in all societies certain behaviours are designated as deviant or rule-breaking and that, for some reason never fully explained, a subset of these rule-breaking behaviours are labelled 'crazy'. It is further asserted that once a person is labelled as mad, he is locked into a stereotyped role and continues to behave according to social expectations of 'madness'. These two assertions are offered as a comprehensive explanation for the entire range of mental illnesses found in all societies. It has never been explained by the social labelling theorists how people who do not know how to act in socially appropriate roles in the first place and are unable to behave according to normal social expectations become so proficient in sensing, learning and performing the deviant role that society suddenly expects of the 'insane'. If they are so adept at conforming to the roles assigned by society to the insane, imitating the conduct expected of those to be judged as cases of schizophrenic or manic illness, why could they not have learned socially appropriate roles in the first place? The mystery is left unresolved.

It is also claimed that, in the absence of an organized professional group created for the purpose of designating specific forms of deviant behaviour as insane, there would be no such thing as mental illness. To sustain such a claim, present-day Western practices would have to be shown to have been in operation at every stage of human history in a wide range of societies, classes and cultures. A general conspiratorial theory would be needed, supported by evidence that only those societies that required internal scapegoats differentiated certain forms of deviant behaviour and singled them out as insanity or mental illness. Furthermore there would be no reason to expect that the actual patterns of behaviour so designated and labelled in different societies would resemble each other.

The main question we wish to examine in this chapter is whether there is worldwide evidence of psychoses existing independently of professional psychiatric labelling. We also need to determine exactly how psychoses manifest themselves, how they are recognized by each society, and how those designated as mentally ill are treated, in terms of healing procedures as well as social role and responses. The evidence from every authoritative source is unequivocal. Psychoses exist and are recognized in all societies that have been studied in depth.[1] The studies of the Eskimo of northwest Alaska and the Yoruba of rural Nigeria by J. Murphy[2] and of the Laotians by Westermeyer[3] are perhaps the most germane for our theme. These two workers investigated societies not influenced by Western psychiatric practitioners or values. They did not try to diagnose psychoses by Western standards, but rather tried to determine, by means of systematic observation, which persons were considered mentally ill by the local population and how this judgement was reached. Murphy concluded that patterns of disturbed thought and behaviour closely similar to schizophrenia were found among the Eskimo and Yoruba, and that the condition was sufficiently distinctive and noticeable for a name to have been created for it in each society. Similarly, Westermeyer found a core group of thirty-five persons within twenty-seven Laotian villages who were considered *ba* (insane) by the villagers.[4] At the time of this study there were no practising psychiatrists or psychiatric institutions in Laos.

The Eskimo word for 'being crazy' is *nuthkavihak*. The Behaviours associated with *nuthkavihak* are as follows:

talking to oneself, screaming at someone who does not exist, believing that a child or husband was murdered by witchcraft when nobody else believes it, believing oneself to be an animal, refusing to eat for fear eating will kill one, refusing to talk, running away, getting lost, hiding in strange places, making strange grimaces, drinking urine, becoming strong and violent, killing dogs, and threatening people.[5]

The Yoruba word *were* is translated as insanity. It encompasses the following behaviours:

hearing voices and trying to get other people to see their source though none can be seen, laughing when there is nothing to laugh at, talking all the time or not talking at all, asking oneself questions and answering them, picking up sticks and leaves for no purpose except to put them in a pile, throwing away food because it is thought to contain *juju*, tearing off one's clothes, defecating in public and then mushing around in the feces, taking up a weapon and suddenly hitting someone with it, breaking things in a state of being stronger than normal, believing that an odor is continuously being emitted from one's body.[6]

Murphy comments that indigenous healing practices were used for both *nuthkavihak* and *were*.

Westermeyer described several folk categories of insanity in Laos.[7] The term *ba* (insane, crazy or mad) refers to the following types of behaviour: seeing and hearing things not perceived by others ('They see things in the dirt that are not there, pick them up and examine them even though nothing is in their hand'); having unusual thoughts not validated by others ('They think they are a big or important person even though they are not'); unusual and apparently purposeless or dangerous behaviour ('Some do very foolish things, like throw food out of the house, kill a chicken or a dog, or eat things out of the dirt – even the dung of farm animals'); impaired thought, memory, logic, intelligence ('Their speech does not make any sense; they talk foolishly'). Other behaviours possibly warranting a *ba* label included 'assault upon others, risk to self, destruction of property, other socially disruptive or problematic behaviour, impairment of interpersonal relationships and communication, psychological dysfunction, and certain somatic symptoms'. The designation of someone as *ba* was applied by relatives and fellow villagers. Westermeyer also describes concepts related to *ba*. These include *ba lu at*, characterized by talking foolishly or in a constant or rapid manner and becoming very angry for little or no reason; *ba puang*, referring to an insane wanderer; *ba mu*, referring to people with convulsions. The Laotians also use a term *sia chit*, meaning literally 'lost mind' and translating into English as 'nervous breakdown' or 'emotional disturbance'. *Sia chit* persons complain of constant sadness or crying spells, sleeping difficulties, heavy feelings in the chest and heart, and feelings of weakness.

In a survey of medieval chronicles and saints' lives, Kroll and Bachrach found that references were occasionally made to mentally deranged people.[8] These references to mental illness were never a major focus of the narrative, but occurred in the larger context of a description of sick people coming to a shrine, or being brought to a holy man for a cure, or merely as a noteworthy event which is commented upon and then passed over. No single instance is extensively or systematically described, but if one compiles the common or major features of many descriptions, then a composite picture emerges of what behaviours were considered insane by family and villagers in Europe in the Middle Ages. These include the following: losing one's wits; losing one's reason; babbling; refusing to speak; being unaware of where one is; wandering aimlessly; neglect of self, especially food and clothing; living wild in the forest and wearing animal skins; howling like a beast; thrashing about; raging; throwing stones at others; violent assaults upon others; biting everything to shreds; tearing oneself to pieces with one's own teeth.

This list of behaviours is remarkably similar to those described by J. Murphy and Westermeyer and reflects the folk concepts and understandings of mental illness, not, we again emphasize, a medical notion imposed by a professional group. Cases of insanity were recognized as such by family and neighbours because the behaviours were by and large bizarre and made up a pattern that resembled no other pattern. The insanity label was not conferred lightly and, as Westermeyer especially points out,[9] there were available to the villagers a series of lesser concepts and terms that could be used to describe minor conditions which we would consider to be in the neurotic range.

Complementing such naturalistic studies is an extensive series of clinical studies of indigenous populations in which Western psychiatric criteria are used to identify mentally ill persons. The most extensive project of this type is that sponsored by the World Health Organization – the International Pilot Study of Schizophrenia which investigated 1202 psychotics (without other organic diseases) in nine countries (China (Taiwan), Columbia, Czechoslovakia, Denmark, India, Nigeria, United Kingdom, the United States and the USSR).[10] The aims of this pilot study were to investigate: (1) in what sense schizophrenic disorders can be said to exist in different parts of the world, (2) whether there are groups of schizophrenic patients with similar characteristics in every one of the countries studied, (3) whether there are groups of schizophrenics whose symptoms differ from one country to another, and (4) whether the clinical course of schizophrenia differs between countries. The methodological goal was to determine whether a collaborative international study using uniform assessment questionnaires and uniform diagnostic criteria was even feasible. The conclusions were that schizophrenic disorders existed in all the countries studied and that there was a high degree of similarity between the centres with regard to the symptoms that occur most frequently in their schizophrenic patients. The symptoms that identified a core group of schizophrenics in all the centres were delusions, hallucinations, and blunted and constricted emotional display.

The overall findings of the WHO pilot project provided supporting evidence that schizophrenia indeed occurs all over the world and that its main features are similar in each country. However, there were some discordant data derived from the follow-up studies of these patients, as well as more impressionistic data from other studies, that raise questions about the extent of the effect of cultural influences upon the symptomatology and course of schizophrenia. Studies by Rin and Lin of Formosan aborigines and Chinese in Formosa,[11] by H. B. M. Murphy and Raman in Mauritius,[12] by Waxler in Sri Lanka,[13] and by Torrey et al. in Papua New Guinea[14] all report a lower incidence of schizophrenia amongst native populations with minimal contact with industrialized and urbanized people as compared with natives with more contact. Murphy and Raman also found that schizophrenic illnesses in Mauritius followed a more benign course than similar-type illnesses in England and Wales. The more systematic WHO follow-up study supported these findings: the course of the schizophrenic illness was more benign in the non-industrialized countries, most notably Nigeria and India. The fact that the course and outcome of schizophrenia, as of other disorders, are affected by familial and social factors is well-established, and does not in itself alter the validity of the concept of the disease.

With regard to the similarity of schizophrenic symptoms in different cultures, H. B. M. Murphy has reviewed anecdotal and impressionistic studies from the work of forty psychiatrists in twenty-seven countries.[15] There are differences in the symptomatology across cultures, although apparently not enough to make the schizophrenic illness unrecognizable as such. Thus, paranoid illnesses are seen more frequently in urban populations; religious delusions in Christian populations, and less frequently in Buddhist, Hindu and Shintoist populations; catatonic symptoms least frequently in Euro-American populations; delusions of grandeur most frequently in rural populations; and social withdrawal most frequently in Japanese and Okinawans.

Furthermore, several studies have been made to determine whether schizophrenic symptoms change in the course of time in the same culture. Varga compared case records from Budapest hospitals from 1910 and 1960 and documented some variations across time and two world wars, such as an increase in paranoid symptoms and a decrease in florid symptomatology.[16] He concluded, however, that the similarities were more striking than the differences in the picture of schizophrenia in the two time periods. It is also possible that these reported differences may merely represent variations in the manifestations of the disease, just as the sequelae of group A haemolytic streptococcal infections may variously include rheumatic fever (cardiac involvement), acute glomerulonephritis (kidney involvement) and Sydenham's chorea (brain involvement), in addition to the usual disease picture of fever and joint pains.

It must be emphasized that in all these studies there are serious methodological difficulties regarding selection of patients, gathering of information, and arrangement and interpretation of data. And there may be observer bias regarding symptoms because one is predisposed to organize one's observations along culturally defined lines, ignoring discrepant findings. The WHO study was the most scrupulous in attempting to avoid these errors, and here the evidence supports the notion that schizophrenia is found worldwide but takes a more benign course in non-industrialized countries. But even in this study there may have been a sampling error such that the patients from industrialized countries were already, at the beginning of the study, in a more advanced and chronic stage of their illness than their non-industrialized counterparts. Complex as the facts may be, they are impossible to reconcile with themes of labelling or the systematic invalidation of those who may pose a threat to the established order by agents such as psychiatrists appointed for this purpose. They are consistent only with the existence of some universally prevalent disorder rooted in biological factors though shaped by contingencies of personality development and familial and social influences.

4 A consideration of the mind–body problem and its bearing on the concept of disease

There appear to be two separate lines of attack on psychiatry which are often merged to appear as one. One attack is based on social and political grounds, alleging that the psychiatric profession functions in society as an instrument of the 'power structure', simultaneously enhancing its own influence and material comfort.

Many of the arguments used to support this attack on psychiatry's socio-political role depend upon a second line of attack, that is, the attack against the scientific legitimacy of psychiatry.[1] This consists first of an accusation that psychiatry has 'medicalized' essentially (non-medical) deviant behaviour by the very acts of diagnosis and treatment, and second of the contrary assertion that there are no such conditions as mental illness. The antipsychiatry writers are obliged by their ideological commitments, rather than by consideration of what mentally ill persons are really like, to assert that mental illnesses are not illnesses.

For some critics of capitalist society, it is convenient to blame the evils of capitalism for the existence of mental illness. But such a standpoint must be rooted strictly in a wholly environmental theory of causation which ignores the contribution of genetics, metabolic abnormalities, and even biological variability and vulnerability. That such theoretical gymnastics are not inherent in the nature of Marxist reasoning is clear from the concept of mental illness in contemporary China. There, dialectical materialism prevails but the environment is not blamed for the occurrence of mental illness. Kleinman has reported, on the basis of his studies at Hunan Medical College, that the major, and almost the only, explanations of mental illnesses put forward in China are biological, mainly neurological.[2] But for some critics of bourgeois society the political capital that can be made from the presence of mentally ill persons once biological factors in causation have been dismissed proves irresistible.

The viewpoint about mental illnesses that is used by some Marxists to support their ideology is advanced by Szasz to reach quite opposite political conclusions. One can march to the right or left on common ground. Szasz's libertarian principles are rescued from grappling with the hard medical and social problems of insanity defence, criminal responsibility and civil commitment by denying that mental illness exists at all.

In this chapter we will examine the basis in philosophy for the claim that mental illnesses are not illnesses. We will, in the following chapter, examine the basis in

45

medical knowledge for this same claim. If these claims are found wanting, then the trappings of philosophical and medical justification will have been stripped from the political arguments of Szasz and the other labelling theorists. At that point it will have to be acknowledged (as Moore has written), 'that mental illness is not a myth but a cruel and bitter reality that has been with the human race since antiquity'.[3] We can examine Szasz's social policy of not inferfering with the suicidal intentions of depressed and schizophrenic persons and the homicidal intentions of paranoid persons. We can examine on his own terms whether such policies, and the related criticisms of present psychiatric approaches to the mentally ill, stand up as credible and reasonable.

Szasz's argument alleges that illnesses can be separated into the 'mental' and 'physical', and that 'mental' illnesses do not resemble 'physical' illnesses closely enough to be considered 'real' illnesses. The argument proceeds that illnesses, to be illnesses, must have a demonstrable bodily lesion, such as a broken arm or a tubercular-infected lung. Furthermore the method of diagnosis of 'physical' illnesses is said to consist in discovering the pathology in the diseased organ. The subject matter of psychiatry, it is alleged, consists of behaviours which are judged to be deviant by others who do not behave in that manner. Diagnosis consists not in finding a pathological organ, but in labelling certain forms of deviant behaviour as illnesses. Thus Szasz is willing to regard 'as diseases only those processes occurring in the body (human or animal) which they [the physicians] can identify, measure, and demonstrate in an objective, physico-chemical manner'.[4] Accordingly, there must be disease present in the tissues – 'histopathological change', as he terms it. Leifer similarly states, 'The criteria for medical disease are physicochemical, while the criteria for psychiatric disease are social and ethical. To diagnose and treat physical disorders we use methods of physics and chemistry. To identify and eliminate mental disorders we use methods of social communication, evaluation, and influence'.[5]

The critics of psychiatry do not appear to be too much embarrassed by their off-handed manner of referring to psychotic behaviours as rule-breaking behaviour. The social labelling theorists, for example, want it both ways – that the deviant behaviour is both trivial and glaring. They state that initially a person behaves a little peculiarly. This peculiar behaviour comes to be labelled by a psychiatrist (or other health professional) as an illness such as schizophrenia. Once the individual concerned has been so stigmatized, he proceeds to behave in accordance with the psychiatrist's preconceptions of 'schizophrenic' behaviour. The small deviance becomes a large deviance just in response to the alleged social expectations, with no reference to the individual's psychological or biological contributions to these processes.

Szasz does not advance any theory of deviant behaviour. He merely asserts that a certain percentage of human beings will act strangely and rejects the illness model as an explanation of such behaviour. He is willing to acknowledge that brain disease may cause someone to act peculiarly, in which case we should not call it 'mental' illness. But if there is no demonstrable brain disease, there is no illness.

Relevance of the mind–body problem

The consideration of mind–body relationships is not an esoteric subject, for it forms one of the major grounds for attacking the concept of psychiatry as a branch of medicine. If medicine is concerned with the study and care of diseases, and if diseases are only of the body (abnormality of anatomical structure or physiological function), and if the mind is completely separate and different from the body, then there can be no diseases, and no medicine, of the mind. The entire argument rests upon a specific dualist solution to the mind–body problem.

The relation of mind to body constitutes an issue of central importance in the life sciences. It poses refractory conceptual difficulties and endless dilemmas. If we think we understand what material things are (chairs, tables, grass, insects, individual people), how are we to understand and make verifiable inferences about mind, a non-material thing? The very term 'thing' designates a material reality. If we accept in an uncritical layman's sense that people do 'have' minds, or that each person has one 'mind', how can this mind, a non-material something, influence a body, a material thing, and how can the body influence the mind? How can one's mind, whatever it is, 'tell' one's body what to do? Perhaps 'mind' is an illusion, and there exist only bodies. Does this mean that, at least at a behavioural level, there is no free will, that this too is an illusion? And if there are only bodies, not minds, how is it that one is aware of oneself? I think, I contemplate, I suffer, I enjoy, I plan, I feel anger, I remember. As Descartes pointed out, one has, or appears to have, direct evidence for one's persistent existence, continuing through time and space. The inability of philosophy or science to explain how such perceptions and experiences can occur reflects a failure to arrive at a satisfactory solution of the mind–body problem. A logical or scientific 'proof' that a mind cannot exist would appear to be absurd from a subjective point of view. In this context, Searle points out that four features – consciousness, intentionality, subjectivity and mental causation – are intrinsically characteristic of mental states and, as he phrases it, 'if your theory ends up by denying any one of them, you know you have made a mistake somewhere'.[6] Yet, arguing convincingly that the existence of mental states cannot be dismissed still leaves unanswered the nature of the mind–body relationship.

Perhaps, as many contemporary philosophers have suggested, the mind–body problem is really a pseudo-problem, erected upon a deceptive foundation of loose and imprecise language.[7] Thus, if we would refine our use of the word 'thing' we would see that mind and body are not 'things' of the same logical type; and if we would refine our use of the word 'cause' we would not wonder how the non-material mind can 'cause' the material body to move and thus violate the laws of physics. We might even come to understand that because we have a word for a thing, we cannot assume that the thing exists. Rorty discusses this issue by way of an analogy with witches and demons.[8] There was a time when people believed in witches and called certain kinds of women witches, and certain kinds of men, sorcerers. We now understand that there are no witches or sorcerers, as far as we can tell, and that the actions (accidents, storms, cattle disease) which were attributed to them must be explained by other mechanisms. We can still use the term 'witch' and understand what is meant, but we no longer claim that witches are real things. In a similar manner, we can use the term 'mind' and know what is meant, but not assume that minds are real things. Rorty goes even further and states that psychological states, such as sensations, may not exist. When we speak of 'pains', we are really referring to brain processes or, more specifically, to neuronal activity in C-fibres, thalamus and sensory cortex. Rorty acknowledges that the claim that there is no such thing as a sensation (or a mind) seems scandalous, just as a putative witch might be scandalized if told witches do not exist. However, Rorty argues that this 'intuitive implausibility' rests solely on the fact that the elimination of mentalistic terms (mind, sensation, feel) from our vocabulary would be impractical – nothing more.

There is much merit to this argument, and certainly a clarification of our many uses of language would help to eliminate considerable misunderstandings and logically invalid arguments. But somehow all the linguistic analyses in the world do not seem to eliminate totally the persistent questions of how one comes to have consciousness, whether the 'I' that one senses has a real existence, and how all one's 'mental processes' relate to one's brain processes. There are additional questions that are less amenable to rational discussion and scientific proof, such as whether the mind will persist beyond bodily death, whether the mind can leave the body, whether 'mental activity' can exert physico-chemical forces at a distance, such as bending spoons or moving objects; and whether minds can communicate with each other independently of our usual bodily means.[9]

Historical perspectives

Although there has always been awareness of a distinction between mind (or soul) and body in Western consciousness, the nature of this distinction was radically altered in the seventeenth century by the writings of Descartes (1596–1650) and others. Before the Renaissance, mind and body were thought of as composing a unity. It is not that Descartes and his scientific contemporaries thought mind and body were not a unity. However, the new seventeenth-century notion of the body as a complex machine loosened the linkage between mind and body. Thereafter, each was imagined as able to function without the other. Mind, as the principle of reason, could function without body. And body, as a machine following mechanical principles, could move and be active without mind. In fact, it was conceded that mind was not necessary as an explanation of complex animal behaviour. It was only in humans, and only because of the function of reason, that the existence of a mind was retained by Descartes. Hobbes, however, carried this line of thinking to its next logical conclusion, which is that if animal behaviour is explicable by mechanistic principles without resort to mind, so too is human behaviour, including reason.[10] Imagination is just the after-effects of decaying sensation, motivation is the last motion in a sequence of motions, and decision is the unfolding of our natural drive to self-preservation. This degree of separability of mind and body, and the question of the existence of mind, was a creation of the new scientific mentality and has informed and guided the development of medical thinking over the past three centuries.[11]

However, the deeper roots of Western culture did not subscribe to the mind–body split known as Cartesian dualism. The two major sources of the Christian world-view, the Judaic and Greek traditions, held to a unitary concept of the person. The Old Testament particularly treats soul and body as one and does not really advance the notion of a soul surviving the death of the body. Hankoff has pointed out that although the ancient Israelites had terms for soul, emotion and possibly mind, as well as terms for the parts of the anatomy, these terms 'do not suggest a division of the individual into a mental and physical reality but rather serve as designations for various functions of the psychophysical unity'.[12]

Much of Greek philosophical thought is preoccupied with mind–body considerations. Several of the Platonic dialogues (*Phaedo, Phaedrus, Timaeus*, parts of the *Republic*) take up in detail the puzzling relations between mind (soul) and body. Although no single unifying statement is to be found that resolves these dilemmas, there is prevalent in Platonic thought the concept of an immortal soul (and of individual souls) which is different from and superior to the body. The concept of a functioning body *without* a soul is impossible. The relationship between the two is complex: the soul itself is composed of three 'parts' (rational, willing, appetitive) with each part having special ties with particular parts of the body. As Van Peursen points out, Plato's dualism is not 'primarily a matter of ontological theory, but is ethico-religious in character'.[13] Plato is concerned to examine the implications of mind–body relations for the ethical foundations and prescriptions of human conduct, not merely to speculate about the ultimate composition of the universe.

In a similar way, in the period from the fall of Rome to the beginning of the Renaissance, thinkers were much preoccupied with mind–body questions, and the world-view within which these questions were framed provided the starting point for post-Renaissance thinking. The puzzle of the relationship of incorporeality to corporeality appeared in debates about angels and about what is the moment in the process of dying at which the soul leaves the body. It also appeared in debates about matters of more practical importance – as, for example, the ways in which the bodily passions interfere with the attainment of true spirituality.[14]

However, with the rise of a scientific mentality in the sixteenth and seventeenth centuries, people became aware, as Putnam describes, 'that the physical world is strikingly causally closed'.[15] There was also a shift away from the qualitative thinking of the medieval world, in which almost anything could exert an influence on almost anything else, towards a quantitative mode of thought that demanded adherence to materialistic notions of causality.

The mind–body crisis of the seventeenth century, exemplified by the writings of Descartes and Hobbes, lay relatively dormant for the next two centuries. The discoveries of physics and chemistry were not applicable to the elucidation of the 'machinery' of the body until the early twentieth century. Since then, the rapid development of the brain sciences, and their merger with a range of disciplines from psychiatry and psychology to biochemistry, molecular biology and computer science have reawakened the mind–body issues which pressed so urgently upon Renaissance man.

It is important to appreciate that the mind–body problem remains a problem; it has not been resolved or solved, and certainly not by Szasz's few paragraphs or pages. There have been many ingenious and detailed contenders for the honour of solving the apparently unsolvable: epiphenomenalism (consciousness is the result or product of a material process, but can have no effect on matter), parallelism (states of consciousness and brain processes run parallel with one another, but neither can affect the other), interactionism (mind and brain interact with each other, although they are different), ordinary language (there is no real problem; our conceptual confusion derives from an imprecise and misleading use of language), and identity theory (mental states, such as sensations, thoughts and ideas are identical with brain processes).[16]

Most philosophers and brain researchers think that the evidence supports a materialistic identity theory with little basis for a mind–body dualism. However, there are distinguished philosophers, including Karl Popper, and neurophysiologists, including the Nobel prize recipient John Eccles, who argue, from the evidence, for the separate existence of mind.[17] Eccles, particularly, has put forward the view that the location of the interaction between mind and brain (not the location of mind) is in some of the association areas of the left (dominant) cerebral cortex.[18]

However, not one of these theories, either materialistic or dualistic, has succeeded in answering the pointed criticisms addressed to them, or in convincing the philosophically sceptical that the solution really solves anything. Schopenhauer referred to the mind–body problem as the riddle of the universe (*Weltknoten*, literally world-knot).[19]

Neurosciences and the mind–body problem

Although the philosophical problem as to the nature of the relationship between consciousness (and other mental processes, if such exist) and brain processes has remained controversial through the centuries, there has been an accumulation of factual information relevant to mind–brain 'interactions', particularly over the past hundred years. This information is based upon the findings of psychiatry, psychology and the neurosciences. In general terms, it links more closely mental activity to brain processes. Thus the functional mapping of the cerebral cortex (and subcortical structures) has established specific anatomical regions and connections which subserve particular activities (speech, memory, spatial orientation, appetite, wakefulness) and which, if damaged, lead to an alteration of function. The microstructure of the synapse has been somewhat elucidated beyond the simple recognition of a chemical mediator to a richer understanding of the many chemical neurotransmitters involved, the importance of receptor sites, and the quantitative relationships between production, release, removal and storage of these biochemical factors.[20] And there are a number of findings that show one cannot speak of mental processes, as we know them, independently of a neurological substructure: the recent discovery of endorphins,[21] the internally produced narcotic-like chemicals which may in the future raise important philosophical issues regarding voluntary versus determined behaviour; the increased awareness and demonstration (albeit oversimplified) of the differential functioning of the two cerebral hemispheres, with logical-linguistic left hemispheric functions contrasting with holistic-spatial right hemispheric functions;[22] the preliminary demonstration of some biochemical abnormalities that seem to be correlated both with states of depression and with schizophrenic illnesses;[23] the unequivocal demonstration of an important genetic component in schizophrenia, mood disorders, and even personality traits;[24] and the recognition of hormonal influences on mood and thinking.

This does not provide evidence for an identity between mental states and brain processes and therefore does not support a strictly reductionistic-materialistic solution which would claim, as J. J. C. Smart does, that 'man is a vast arrangement of physical particles, but there are not, over and above this, sensations or states of consciousness'.[25] But it does argue, by linking mental activity so intimately and inextricably to brain processes, against a dualistic viewpoint that posits an existence of mind independent of body.

Although the argument often seems esoteric, the fact is that the theoretical and the practical implications are great. As Eccles writes in the preface to Polten's refutation of scientific materialism,

if Feigl (identity theory) is right, then man is no more than a superior animal, entirely a product of the chance and necessity of evolution. His conscious experiences, even those of the most transcendent creative and artistic character, are *nothing but* the products of special states of the neural machinery of his brain, itself a product of evolution. If Polten is right, man has in addition a supernatural component, his conscious self that is centered on his pure ego. Thus with his spiritual nature he transcends the evolutionary origin of his body and brain, and in so far could participate in immortality.[26]

The corollary of contemporary dualism is the survival of the concept of free will and with it the notion of individual responsibility; the corollary of scientific materialism is determinism, with only the subjective appearance but not the reality of free will. The possibility of determinism and its twin, reduced (or absence of) responsibility, touches at the very core of many of the objections to the medical model of psychiatry. For once a small degree of determinism is allowed, there appears to be no way of avoiding the extension of this to the very end of its logical road: man's actions are the product of neural wiring, hormonal and biochemical shifts, alterations in the cellular structures (gross brain injury to submicroscopic particles) and physiology. If major alterations in brain activity undeniably influence or absolve responsiblity for aberrant (such as criminal) behaviours, then might not the same be said for smaller alterations, and even smaller alterations, and so forth?

It becomes clear why the mind–body problem plays such a critical role in the attack on or defence of a medical model of psychiatry. The attack on psychiatry rests on the assumption that the mind–body problem has been solved by dualism, and in a simplistic manner at that. This solution involves a separation of the mental and physical, sharp enough to allow thought and behaviour to proceed in the absence of a neural substructure and physiology, and to allow physiology to proceed uninfluenced by mental activities. Such a viewpoint ignores the accumulated evidence pointing to the inseparability of brain (body) states and mental states, especially in conditions of illness.

In an effort to accommodate the weakness of the argument that equates disease with structural lesions, the notion of illness is expanded by Szasz and others to include altered physiological functioning. But once altered functioning is brought into consideration, then the boundaries between physiology and psychology become obscured.

There is a physiology of normal gastric functioning, just as there is a physiology of normal mental functioning. The physiology of gastric functioning is certainly not as complex as the brain processes which underlie mental functioning, but neither is it as simple as most people probably assume. Gastric functioning involves well-known biochemical processes: the production, storage and release of enzymes that digest or break down different food constituents; the prevention of autodigestion of the mucosal lining of the stomach by the secretion of protective mucus and the constant regeneration of new layers of gastric cells; the selective absorption of particular nutrients and the prevention of absorption of other nutrients, such as undigested protein segments which would stimulate antibody formation in the blood and lymphatic systems; the regulation of blood supply to the gut; the integration of gut activity (peristalsis), liver and gall bladder activity, and food-seeking behaviour requiring higher neural activity; and the production by the gut of a hormone which signals satiety to the brain.[27] All these activities and many more comprise normal gastric functioning. Abnormal gastric functioning occurs when one or more elements of this integrated activity malfunction.

The analogy with the brain must be obvious. The functioning of the nervous system is infinitely more complex, and what we understand of its complexities is infinitesimal when we compare it with what we do not understand. Nevertheless, a reasonable amount is known and knowledge is increasing very rapidly. When some of the physiology underlying mental activity is known, it is likely that we will perceive that the distinctions between normal and abnormal brain functioning may be quite small. This is illustrated by the differential levels in health and disease of the metabolites of the neurotransmitter serotonin that are found in the cerebrospinal fluid. A normal serotonin level permits normal mood maintenance. An abnormally low level, probably reflecting more basic disturbances of biochemical enzyme regulation, seems to cause, or is accompanied by, severe depression with suicidal preoccupation.[28]

This type of analogy may be very offensive to those who prefer to think about the mysteries of life and the existential meanings of joy and despair. We do not mean to disparage such views. But this does not weaken the observation that as the neurosciences elucidate brain mechanisms more fully and the gaps in the continuum between normal and abnormal functioning are filled in, the distinctions which Szasz tries to make between abnormal behaviour caused by gross brain disease and 'deviant behaviour' in which there are no observable lesions but which may prove to be related to specific alterations in complex neural subsystems will be seen as spurious or non-existent.

Is increased gastric secretion and the sensation of characteristic 'peptic ulcer' pain, in the absence of X-ray evidence of a duodenal ulcer, to be considered a peptic ulcer nevertheless? If the increased gastric secretion is indubitably linked to times of emotional stress, should the 'mental' component be considered part of the illness? If altered gastric secretion and stomach pain are considered an illness, why not altered (incoherent) thinking following chronic use of amphetamines or LSD? And if altered thinking following amphetamine use is accepted as an illness, why not altered thinking in the absence of amphetamine use? Is it that we believe that we can measure gastric secretions more accurately (certainly not more easily) than altered thinking? It is not even clear why the person with stomach pain (but no indubitable proof of an ulcer) should consider himself as being ill just on the basis of having pain.

How did such social conventions ever arise? And if pain, which is a subjective or mental experience, is enough to convince one person that he is ill, in what sense does this differ from a feeling of depression, also a subjective experience, which convinces another person that he is ill? It can only be that it is not the presence of a bodily lesion that is the universal criterion of illness, but rather the perception and character of pain (whether physical or emotional) or dysfunction (whether physical or mental).

There is a tendency to define diseases in terms of the prevailing technologies.[29] With the development of the autopsy as an investigative procedure, disease in its gross pathological forms could be identified. It was recognized that clinical patterns of symptoms in life could be associated with the pathological finding at autopsy. With the development of the microscope, disease in its cellular form, as well as certain infectious agents (bacteria, but not viruses) could be recognized, and so on with the development of biochemical, autoimmune and electron microscopical techniques. This analogy could be extended to psychological measurement techniques, which are as reliable as many 'physical' techniques. It is not clear that levels of gastric hydrochloric acid measure 'stomach function' in a way that is essentially different from that in which a depression scale measures 'brain function' (taking brain function here to signify the final end organ expression of the entire biopsychosocial complex that constitutes depressive states). After all, the stomach has many functions, of which the secretion of 'proper' amounts of hydrochloric acid at 'proper' times is only one; it has been established that excess acid secretion is associated with gastric irritation and that insufficient gastric secretion is associated with pernicious anaemia. Mood regulation is one function of the brain, and a mood scale which measures intensity of perceived sadness can reliably reflect an overall condition of depression.

In view of the increasing sophistication of measurement of all bodily functions, it seems that the critical task would be to decide – on both medical and psychological grounds – exactly what criteria should be used in making the distinction between health and sickness. If we do not do this, we must be prepared to consider seriously Sackett's definition of normality: 'a normal person is anyone who has not been sufficiently investigated'.[30]

Before discussing the concept of disease, it might serve well to review briefly what ground we have covered so far. We have outlined the main arguments in the controversies surrounding the status of psychiatry as a legitimate branch of medicine, and regarding the question of whether mental diseases are forms of illness or socially deviant forms of conduct devoid of kinship with disease and illness in the medical sense of these terms. We have stated our basic position that these complex problems do not permit of simple solutions, that there are few if any sharp dividing lines in nature between health and illness, and that the evidence from historical, cross-cultural and medical studies does not support the arguments of antipsychiatry writers. We have shown that a concept of insanity has existed in all historical periods and societies investigated, that medical practitioners have always included mental disturbances as a form of illness, and that the predominant theory of causation of mental illness throughout the history of Western civilization has been anatomical and physiological, not supernatural or demonological. We have cited cross-cultural studies which demonstrate that persons with conditions similar to the Western concept of schizophrenia are found in non-industrial societies which have not been exposed to psychiatric influences. Finally, we have discussed the complexity of the mind–body controversy, and have pointed out that this 'riddle of the universe' remains unresolved and that the dualistic viewpoint to which the antipsychiatry writers attach so much importance is merely one proposal from a whole range of proposals – and one which it would be particularly difficult to verify or refute.

5 Medical and alternative models of mental disease

There is no official or authoritative medical model, either for psychiatry or for any other discipline within the field of medicine. A model, any model, is a proposal for organizing the way we look at and understand complex phenomena. Models are merely useful and do not make claims to be true or false. Especially in its early stages, it is more important that a model should be capable of incorporating the known facts, of accommodating findings seemingly at variance with it, and be open to challenge by fresh evidence. All scientific models, including those inherent in systems of psychiatric classification and diagnosis, consist of a series of interrelated hypotheses regarding the phenomena they seek to explore and understand. The subject matter itself cannot be initially circumscribed, for as the model develops, areas previously included might be judged irrelevant and thus excluded, while other areas that were totally unknown or unimaginable emerge as critically important and must be incorporated.

Thus a knowledge of astrology, for over 1500 years considered essential to the diagnostic and therapeutic equipment of the scientific physician, is now regarded as archaic and irrelevant. The scientific model of human health and disease no longer includes the influence of heavenly bodies upon the birth, well-being, attributes and diseases of mankind. However, by contrast, the investigation and understanding of receptor sites, the structures on cell membranes which accept specific molecules as a lock accepts a key, and thereby appear to initiate specific cellular mechanisms, now appears to be a fruitful area of study. This shift in our vision from the cosmic and universal to the submicroscopic and specific is a hallmark of modern science. It can be viewed as symbolic of the diminution of transcendental values, of a loss of any perspective that looks beyond the mechanical – a loss of our sense of beauty and poetry. But, as one result, fewer children die at an early age of infectious diseases, diabetes or congenital defects.

Since the concept of disease itself derives from a model of human health and behaviour, it follows that there exist no such 'things' as diseases. Pneumonia or cancer or hypertension do not exist; instead there are individual persons who have an infected lung, or a malignant growth of the pancreas, or a certain type of circulatory dynamics in the cardiovascular system. It is a convenience for us to speak of pneumonia, cancer and hypertension when we really mean the classes of persons who have these conditions. However the convenience is much greater than merely a linguistic one; the use of disease terms enables us to classify persons and their conditions on the basis of similar and dissimilar features. There are those who object to the classification of humans in any manner whatsoever, claiming that each individual is unique and unclassifiable. Such a statement is clearly illogical, for persons are classified according to what they have in common, and not what is unique.

Classification is a basic biological function, not a procedure invented by statisticians and entomologists.[1] An animal or plant could not survive if it did not discriminate between beneficial and noxious substances. Even a single-celled organism, such as an amoeba, in 'learning' to move towards food or away from an acid solution, is exhibiting an ability to classify, although, it is assumed, not at a self-conscious level. The discriminatory power of the classification scheme appears suited to the needs of the classifier: thus Eskimos have more than a score of terms to describe (and thereby classify) types of snow, and wine connoisseurs have a multitude of terms to describe (and thereby classify) wines.

In medicine the prime, and possible sole, justification for developing classificatory systems is their fruitfulness. In order to know that a person has a type of pneumonia that will be cured by penicillin, one must first recognize that it belongs to the class of pulmonary disease caused by bacteria which will be killed by penicillin. To arrive at the point where a complex medical problem could be formulated in such a simple statement (an example of what we take for granted in modern medicine) has required thousands of years of collaborative human endeavour, including the development of a range of intricate and increasingly precise classificatory schemas (bacteriology, clinical diagnostics, pharmacology), and provides an example of the fruitfulness of a medical approach. Similarly, in order to know that a person has a depression of the class that responds to tricyclic antidepressant medication, one must recognize it by its signs (early morning awakening, weight loss, altered cortisol metabolism) and symptoms (feelings of sadness, lack of energy and interest, poor concentration, thoughts of suicide).

This is tangible progress in the amelioration of human suffering and in the return of ill persons to active, functioning lives. We are not endorsing a teleological theory of human progress in which all past events are evaluated in accordance with how well they contributed to achieving our present advanced state. Nor are we presenting the accomplishments of recognition, classification and treatment of diseased individuals and populations as the apotheosis of two million years of evolving mankind, nor yet suggesting that medical achievements come without spiritual and material cost. Many may prefer to die at home amongst, it is to be hoped, family and friends, rather than in a modern hospital with all sorts of tubes entering and emerging from the anticipated cadaver. But there is little virtue in suffering from and dying of streptococcal pneumonia when penicillin could cure the infection, or dying of an inflamed and ruptured appendix when surgery could cure the condition, or of suffering from a severe melancholia and perhaps committing suicide when electroconvulsive treatments or antidepressant medications could cure the illness. Except for a few rare individuals, living and dying in great pain is not ennobling or uplifting of the soul, especially when treatment is available. Consider these two examples from tenth century northern Europe.

The death of Lothaire, AD 986:
At Laon that same spring, on account of the changing weather, which by the nature of things tends to occur, he began to sicken. Being troubled with the ailment which the physicians call colic, he took to his bed. He had intolerable pains on the right side just above his privates. From the navel to the spleen and thence to the left groin and the rectum, he was stricken with violent pains. His intestines and kidneys were also affected; [he had] constant straining; bloody excretions; at times he lost his voice. Meanwhile he became rigid with the chill of fever. [He had] rumbling of the intestines; constant nausea; vain efforts at belching, swelling of the abdomen, and heart burn . . . at sixty-eight years of age he died.[2] (Richer, Historia, vol III, p. 109)

The death of Count Odo I of Troyes and Chartres, AD 996:
Being troubled by a superfluity of humors, by reason of the change of seasons, he was taken with the ailment which the physicians call synanche. This began on the inside of the throat, and spreading with the rheumatic phlegm settled first in the jaws and cheeks, then in the chest and lungs, with very painful swelling. These parts then became inflamed and feverish, and with the return of the fever on the third day he succumbed to it. Having fallen into this condition, Odo was seized with terrible pains in the throat. The fever in his air passages brought about a stoppage of speech. The trouble did not spread to the top of his head but invaded the midriff and his lungs and liver were afflicted with very acute pain . . . on the fourth day after the beginning of the synanche, Odo died.[3] (Richer, Historia, vol. IV, p. 94)

Such graphic descriptions do serve to remind us of the brutal facts of life and death. We tend either to romanticize or to sterilize illness and dying, forgetting that for the entire history of mankind except for the past hundred years, the slow and agonizing death of sections of the body usually preceded the ultimate death of the person.

Perhaps critics of psychiatry would see it as unfair and illegitimate for psychiatry to share in the credit for the accomplishments of medicine in relieving suffering. But psychiatry is a branch of medicine. The resemblances between psychiatry and other fields of medicine are greater than the differences; the goals, methods, subject matter, ethics and responsibilities are identical. Nevertheless, there are apparent differences which give the semblance of a more profound dichotomy than in fact exists. McHugh and Slavney have provided insight into the nature of the differences:
In the everyday world of the clinic, psychiatrists are distinguished from other medical specialists not because they are concerned with 'minds' rather than 'bodies' but because they focus on complaints appearing in people's thoughts, perceptions, moods and behaviours rather than in their skins, bones, muscles, and viscera . . . The diagnostic process may be simple or difficult, but causal explanations are always complex and depend on the physician's capacity to evaluate issues ranging from intermediary metabolism (a 'body' issue) to interpersonal misunderstanding (a 'mind' issue). Psychiatric concerns thus extend from the ultrastructure of the body to the relationship of groups of minds within a social context.

It is more than the breadth of the field, however, that leads to a special problem in psychiatry. It is that ambiguity represented by the issues of body and mind with which we are struggling. This is a fundamental discontinuity in the hierarchical sequence of psychiatric explanations that makes the relationship between such issues as metabolism and misunderstanding obscure. This discontinuity occurs at what we call the brain–mind junction, a place of uncertain location where suddenly our language describing what we observe changes from talking about tangibles such as cells, neurons, or brains to talking of intangibles such as thoughts, moods, or intentions.[4]

This conceptual limitation in our understanding is not carried over into the pragmatic judgments of the clinical or everyday world. Here it is abundantly clear physical occurrences affect our mental states, that our mental states (thoughts, moods) direct our behaviours and affect our physical states, and that our existence as social beings provides the cultural matrix in which body and mind interact. In this light, it would make sense if the term 'medical model' were to be understood as 'biopsychosocial model'. This is not a linguistic sleight of hand, for no medical model should ignore the psychological and sociological parameters of health and disease. Psychiatrists have in the past few decades directed much effort towards widening and humanizing the perspectives adopted in the theory, practice and teaching of medicine. They have also played a considerable part in the rediscovery and reinstatement of what was at one time a general consensus among the predecessors of this generation of physicians that the whole person – his relationships, talents, successes, griefs and vicissitudes – needs to be taken into account in defining the problem of that person's ill-health and formulating a plan of management.

In fact, even the 'bio' component of the 'biopsychosocial' model must be understood as encompassing an evolutionary concept of biology rather than a narrow mechanistic one. However, the term biopsychosocial is one of those polysyllabic words invented as a corrective when, as a result of specialisation, an unfortunate restrictiveness slowly overtakes a field. Therefore we will continue to use the term medical model, not to indicate ownership of it by the medical profession, but rather to maintain the continuity of its historical roots, which have always been broad-based. We do not need to change its name to accommodate its critics.

Medical models of the past

There are several narrow partial medical models, all of which have reflected particular beliefs or actual technological advances in the understanding of disease in the past. The earliest scientific one is the humoral theory, which held sway for some two thousand years. This postulates that health and disease are the result of the balance or imbalance in the body of the four humours or, more specifically, of the four qualities (hot, cold, dry, moist) of which the humours partake. Anything that could affect the humoral balance, such as weather, food, drink, climate and passions, could affect one's health. The humoral theory was never directly challenged and overthrown; rather it was abandoned, as scientific models generally are, for two interrelated reasons. First, it became too complex and burdensome, as the four qualities themselves were subdivided into degrees and pretended to a precision without having a technology for accurate measurements. Also, it was unfruitful of progress.[5] Therefore, in due course, it was replaced by a newer model. However, although abandoned, the humoral model has left a legacy that is central to all Western concepts of disease, the most obvious of which is the notion of health or disease as reflecting a balance or imbalance in the physiological functioning of the body.

The humoral model was largely replaced by the seventeenth – and eighteenth-century concept of mechanical man. Man was viewed as a complicated, but ultimately understandable machine. Descartes provided the theological legitimacy for this materialistic notion by disengaging the mind–body unity into two separate components, thereby allowing the body to be studied scientifically without worrying about theological implications.

Harvey's revolutionary discovery, published in 1628, of the circulation of the blood in one continuous system, reduced the mystique of blood as the essence of life. As Graubard has written:

What had been presumed to be spirit was actually a fluid, driven through a system of vessels by a rhythmically contracting and dilating organ of muscle tissue, with valves and sluices to aid the flow and joints and mouths to complete the circuit. The picture of the heart as a mechanistic pump controlling the circulation of the blood marked the dawn of scientific materialism in the West.[6]

Newtonian mechanics provided the scientific model for understanding the body. Thus all bodily activities, including life itself, could be explained by the shape, size properties and motions of the particles composing the body fluids, especially blood, and by the properties of the fibrous parts (nerves, vessels, tubules and pores) of the body. The link between mind and brain was mediated by animal spirits, a very fine material substance which communicated the ideas of the mind to the nerves, muscles and glands of the body. Friedrich Hoffman, professor of medicine at the university at Halle and one of the dominant figures in medicine of this period, wrote in 1965:

All philosophers are agreed, that in our machine the first principle of motion is the soul, which you may, if you want, designate as nature, or spirit endowed with mechanical powers, or a most subtle ethereal matter acting in an ordered and specific fashion (I, Chap. III, Sect. 21, p. 12)

. . .

Our body is like a machine which is composed of solid and fluid particles, disposed and arranged in varying order and position (I, Chap. IV, Sect. 1, p. 13).[7]

This application of Newtonian mechanics to life processes represented a revolutionary change in conceptual thinking far removed from the philosophical, teleological and humoral explanations in Aristotelian and scholastic biology. The concept of 'animal spirits' was a necessary scientific thesis at that time in order to bridge the gap between the new findings and older vitalistic beliefs too firmly established to be relinquished all at once. The animal spirits, a material substance, were directly involved in the maintenance of health and the development of illness. Hoffman and his contemporaries did not set apart mental illnesses from all other of man's illnesses. All illnesses were caused by disordered motion of particles.

One hundred years before Pinel removed the chains of the insane and, according to Foucault, before medicine discovered and claimed mental illness, Hoffman wrote the following about disease in general and mental disease in particular:

In the natural state the animal spirits move evenly through the brain, spinal medulla, nerves, and the very delicate fibrillar membranes woven from them. If, however, the motion of these spirits becomes disordered or diminished or fully abolished, very severe diseases arise (I, Chap. VII, Sect. 2, p. 67)

. . .

In melancholics the spirits are indistinct and fixed, and approach a sort of acid nature. They not only leave enduring fixed ideas in the brain pores, but promptly uncover similar traces, of ideas of sadness, terror, fear, and so on (II, Chap. VII, Sect. 49, p. 71)

. . .

In those who are maniacal, the spirits are more sulphurous, raging, and active. Hence, they deposit in the brain ideas that are unstable, and uncover traces similar to themselves (II, Chap. VII, Sect. 50, p. 72)

. . .

Mania can easily pass over into melancholy, and conversely, melancholy into mania. For in either condition the nature of the cerebral pores is damaged, and the fixed acid spirits can readily take on an igneous and sulphurous nature, and can be easily excited by very violent motion (II, Chap. VII, Sect. 52, p. 72)[7]

The mechanical man model did not immediately generate any specific progress in medical diagnosis or treatment but rather provided the substratum upon which the advances of the last two centuries rest. Although some critics may not see the mechanical model as progress, it permitted the detailed investigation of subsystems of the body. Rather than proceeding deductively from the general to the particular, as we do in reasoning from social organization down to individuals, the progress of science is hierarchical from below upwards, i.e. the units of explanation are sought from narrower rather than broader classes of phenomena (except in the rare synthesizing theories such as those of Newton and Einstein). Thus, physics becomes more mathematical, chemistry more physical, biology more biochemical, and sociology more biological. The fact that the units of explanation must delve into smaller and smaller subsystems does not mean that integration of these units into comprehensive and comprehensible organizations will not occur. However, critics of science would have it that only investigation of larger units (populations, social classes, economic forces) can provide 'answers' and can avoid the otherwise inevitable dehumanization caused by the sciences. This is one more ideology which is completely unsupported, and ignores the dynamic nature of science. Thus the mechanical model, convincing as was the eminently logical model in the seventeenth century and its humoral predecessor in its day, was itself incorporated into a broader medical model.[8]

The nineteenth century saw the emergence of medicine as a scientific discipline, a change parallel to that which had occurred in the physical sciences in the centuries before. Koch, working independently but building on the work of Pasteur and others, demonstrated the role of bacteria in the genesis of infectious diseases. He outlined the four conditions necessary to show that bacteria are an aetiological agent of disease. In its restricted form, the infectious disease model focuses on an external agent as the cause of disease, ignoring the host–agent–environment interaction, and serves as the prototype of theories which hold, as Weiner expresses it, 'that most diseases can be explained on the basis of single causes'.[9]

Simultaneously with the development of the infectious disease model came the development of the cellular pathology model. This was the outgrowth of several centuries of investigations into the gross and microscopic pathological anatomy found in diseased organs. On the basis of these findings, Virchow put forward the view that manifest disease is nothing more or less than the anatomical and functional changes that derive from diseased cells and organs.

It is these two nineteenth-century models of disease that are invoked by the critics of psychiatry to support their arguments that psychiatric illnesses are not 'true' diseases, i.e. that psychiatric illnesses do not follow Koch's postulates for infectious diseases or Virchow's criteria for cellular pathology. Their logic is clear: if these two sets of criteria are not met, there can be no disease present.

However, these two models are outdated, not because they are false, but rather because they are incomplete, as one would expect a century-old scientific model to be. They too, like their humoral and mechanical predecessors, have been incorporated into a broader model which we have referred to as a biopsychosocial model. This model, reflecting its development within Western civilization, still postulates that disease resides in the individual, as opposed to possibly the tribe, nation or natural surroundings, but recognizes that the factors that ultimately cause the disease or illness are many and varied in type. Eisenberg has summarized this viewpoint succinctly:[10]

human disease inevitably and always reflects the outcome of the process of interaction between human biology and human social organization, a process in which culture occupies a central position. In this respect, psychiatric disorders constitute a subset of human illnesses that do differ in particular, but not in kind from other illnesses.

For example, in the case of infectious diseases, there are, in addition to the pathogenic bacteria or viruses, a multiplicity of host factors, some 'physical' and some 'psychological'. These include the host's immune system and readiness to respond to the invasion of microbes. Thus, for example, not everyone exposed to tuberculosis develops the disease in its complete form. The state of the immune system depends on the host's genetic constitution, nutritional status, viral infections that may produce an immunodeficiency syndrome, previous exposure to similar microbial pathogens, state of fatigue, state of anxiety, level of morale, presence of depression, recent major life changes, and other 'psychological' factors. No one is surprised that thinking about food can stimulate a flow of gastric juices, that sexual arousal through visual imagery will alter regional blood flow, or that being startled will increase cardiac rate. We also know that states of depression are accompanied by chronically elevated levels of corticosteroids circulating in the body and a disturbance in the 'normal' diurnal variation in cortisone production.[11] Is it too great a leap to hypothesize that production of antibodies or alterations of receptor site sensitivity are also affected by (or accompanied by, to avoid a causal implication) significant changes in mood, cognition or major life events? Much recent evidence points in this direction.[12]

Some diseases appear to have a relatively linear path from causes to effect, although the anatomy and biochemistry may be complex. Most illnesses have a multifactorial and interactive group of causes. Progress in medicine consists in elucidating these causes, including the physiological factors in the aetiology of mental illnesses, the psychological factors in the aetiology of traditional medical illnesses, and the social and cultural factors in the aetiology of both.

Clinical and research models

There is, in addition, a distinction between models used for clinical practice on the one hand and models used for investigation. The clinician has to function across multiple dimensions, initially using his human sensibility, insight and unstructured observation of the context of disease, but ultimately using every available means to alleviate suffering. Yet there is a reciprocal relationship between the roles of clinician and investigator. Observations made in the clinic serve as the starting point for posing questions, but these questions must be broken down into smaller units for scientific inquiry.

For example, the understanding of the sequelae of childhood separation from parents stemmed from observations initially made on forty juvenile thieves. From this clinical observation an entire area of investigation of familial and social pathology was uncovered. The scientific task consisted of identifying a whole range of possible adverse influences emanating from parents, the social environment or both, defining them as precisely as possible and submitting their role and the extent of their contributions to stringent enquiries.

As a second example, the rediscovery of childhood abuse in a clinical framework lays bare in all its horror the extent to which physical abuse and emotional deprivation interact to produce a syndrome called psychosocial dwarfism.[13] In this syndrome the child, living in an abusive environment, shows retardation of growth in stature, intelligence, and maturation of behaviour. This long-term failure of the pituitary gland can be reversed within several weeks simply by moving the child into a hospital or another benign environment.

It is from examples such as these that the inadequacies of traditional medical models are most clearly revealed, and the case made for a biopsychosocial model. However, the biopsychosocial model itself is easier to define in a negative way (i.e. in terms of what it is not), than in a positive manner that does not at the same time appear trite.[14] Thus a biopsychosocial model avoids a reductionist definition of disease as merely altered biochemistry or anatomy. It takes into account, in Engel's terms, 'the patient, the social context in which he lives, and the complementary system devised by society to deal with the disruptive effects of illness'.[15] Engel, who has written extensively about the necessity to move from a biomedical to a biopsychosocial model, describes this process as follows:

The boundaries between health and disease, between well and sick, are far from clear and never will be clear, for they are diffused by cultural, social, and psychological considerations. The traditional biomedical view, that biological indices are the ultimate criteria defining disease, leads to the present paradox that some people with positive laboratory findings are told that they are in need of treatment when in fact they are feeling quite well, while others feeling sick are assured that they are well, that is, they have no 'disease'. A biopsychosocial model which includes the patient as well as the illness would encompass both circumstances. The doctor's task is to account for the dysphoria and the dysfunction which lead individuals to seek medical help, adopt the sick role, and accept the status of patienthood. He must weigh the relative contributions of social and psychological as well as biological factors implicated in the patient's dysphoria and dysfunction as well as in his decision to accept or not accept patienthood and with it the responsibility to cooperate in his own health care.[16]

There are, however, several scientific shortcomings to the biopsychosocial model which serve to remind us that, while it appears so much better than the narrow models of previous generations, it is itself limited by time and culture, and will in turn be incorporated into a richer model. As a basic philosophy that serves to inform the approach to patients in medical and in psychiatric practice, its value and importance are undeniable. But as Engel himself points out, the biopsychosocial model can itself become hardened into a dogma that eschews the scientific method.[17] Such a closure of the model at the level of vague statements that all factors are important and must be taken into account threatens to interfere seriously with the continued progress of medicine. For the observations which are needed to attach appropriate weights to the biological, psychological and social aspects of illness in different types of cases are lacking. And to attach the same weight and clinical significance to all these aspects in all diseases is misconceived.

Let us take the case of Huntington's chorea. The morbid risk in first-degree relatives is 50% and almost 100% of those who carry the gene actually develop the disease. Social and familial factors are of course important since the patient's social and familial role and personal dignity are undermined. There is also the effect of assortative mating, namely a tendency for the choice of mates to be highly selective rather than random. This leads to an accumulation of all types of pathology in a family carrying the gene for Huntington's chorea. But these are secondary consequences and cannot be given the same weight as the underlying disturbances in specific cerebral function which will, in the light of recent advances, probably be proved to be expressable in precise neurochemical terms in the near future.

At the other extreme, the situation is quite different in the case of, let us say, anorexia nervosa, anxiety neurosis, conversion hysteria or transsexualism. Familial, psychological and social factors make a far greater contribution, and hereditary influences a very much smaller one than is the case in Huntington's chorea. Unfortunately, the main impact of the causal agents and the interactions between them will have occurred in the formative stages of the patient's development many years before the illness is presented for treatment in the psychiatric clinic. It is likely that there are engrained patterns of neuronal activity and possibly structural changes in the form of specific synaptic connections in the brain. This is possibly one reason (but not necessarily the only one) why all these disorders prove so resistant to psychotherapy alone.

The case of schizophrenia is different again. Hereditary factors make an indubitable contribution. In this instance, modern techniques of genetic research have made it possible to work out the contribution to variance of the different causal factors, apportioning a high percentage to heredity but a quite substantial role also to familial and environmental factors.[18] As far as social influences are concerned, the great majority of systematic studies have demonstrated that the underprivileged social status of schizophrenics is due to gravitation down the social scale. This may follow the onset of symptoms or it may be a result of the personality disorders already present in many of those who will develop a schizophrenic illness. The adverse social circumstances are consequences rather than aetiological agents – a situation far removed from the state of recidivist delinquency.

The biopsychosocial model as enunciated by Engel and others certainly provides a more imaginative, holistic and compassionate approach to the problems of clinical practice in medicine. As a *general* strategy its importance in this context is undeniable. But from the point of view of advancing knowledge and developing specific therapeutic interventions, its major weakness is a tendency to range every type of disorder – neurotic, psychotic, organic, psychosomatic – side by side as though there were nothing to choose between them in the character of the abnormality or in the nature of the aetiological factors involved. It has mainly heuristic value as a set of hypotheses in relation to different classes of medical disorders, to be investigated along genetic, biochemical, physiological, clinical and psychosocial lines with measurements as precise as the situation permits.

In the meantime, the experienced clinician does his best to take all possible factors into account, to place the known causal agents (including environmental factors) and the therapeutic goals in an order of importance and to concentrate his efforts accordingly. He probably gets it right in a high proportion of cases. But precise knowledge is lacking and it does not serve the cause of the biopsychosocial model to put it forward as a doctrinal truth which resolves the major problems of clinical practice.

This discussion serves to illustrate the point that there is a variety of medical models or, alternatively, if such a thing as a 'medical model' exists, it is a flexible one offering a holistic but rational approach to the multitude of phenomena presented by clinical practice. And having regard to the successes of the medical models in recent decades, we can reasonably expect that clinical practice and the public health approaches to the problems of mental health will acquire a more and more solid factual foundation and thus become more precise and effective. This is because medical models pose clear questions that can be refuted or upheld by scientific investigation.

The implication of the public health model

The general applicability of a biopsychosocial model raises the related problems of how to decide where the boundaries between health and illness should be, and how far down the chain of causality social factors should be included within the legitimate concerns of medicine and public health. Our tendency to view disease as existing within the person interferes with extending the concept of disease to include social, psychological and cultural factors. For example, if lung cancer or cardiovascular disease are under consideration, then aetiology must include risk factors of cigarette smoking, dietary habits, patterns of exercise, and occupational stress and exposure. The contribution of these different factors in the causal networks of different diseases in individuals will vary in importance; they are causal *factors*, not solitary causes. Thus the presence of the *Anopheles* mosquito does not *cause* malaria, in the sense that only the introduction of the *Plasmodium* protozoan into the blood stream and the resultant host response (lysis of blood cells, chills, fever) *causes* or is the disease. But it would be a very poor model of malaria indeed which did not include the life cycle of the mosquito and its relevance to policies of public health.

The problem that arises in all considerations is where to draw the line. As soon as the medical model is broadened beyond the diseased individual to take account of the disease as a risk to the community, the probability demarcation between disease and health becomes a major issue in public health policy. The attempt to prevent and eliminate disease has included in the past such actions as protecting the water supply, ensuring adequate sewerage and sanitation, draining swamps where mosquitoes breed, vaccinating dairy cows, inspecting livestock, insisting on commercial refrigeration for perishable goods, keeping carcinogens out of food, legislating the minimum volume of airspace per person in urban apartments, inspecting food handlers, inspecting vehicles for exhaust pollutants, quarantining persons with certain communicable diseases, enacting child welfare laws, and banning pornographic films in theatres and on television.

It becomes clear that there is lack of agreement on how far the physician should venture into the realms of social change and the political process. Should the physician be concerned with infant nutrition, adequate housing for the elderly, improved training for the handicapped, and nuclear disarmament activities? These issues, which are outside the scope of this book, are noted here because they result from broadening the medical model. However, it is also clear that the public health model sets up conflicts between the recognized health needs of the community and the full expression of individual freedom. The debates involving civil commitment of mentally ill persons are further examples of this basic conflict, and will be discussed in the next chapter.

The incorporation of a public health model into a broadened biopsychosocial medical model poses few problems in areas such as ensuring a sanitary water supply and inoculation against the communicable diseases of childhood. Here a firm consensus has evolved over the years. In a similar way, the broadened medical model poses few problems as to what conditions are and are not diseases in such areas as pneumonia, kidney stone and broken bones. The controversial areas are the newer public health concerns such as fluoridation of drinking water and legislating for clean indoor air. And with these must be included measures concerned with abnormalities of behaviour.

Altered function as the hallmark of disease

We have seen that one major argument of antipsychiatry writers is that real diseases take place in diseased organs whereas so-called psychiatric diseases 'take place' in abnormal or deviant social behaviours.[19] We have also demonstrated that many common diseases (hypertension, narcolepsy, asthma, epilepsy) are manifested as altered function, not structure. In fact with a few exceptions (such as skin rashes and broken bones) the delineation of a disease – that is the description of the clinical syndrome, its course and its treatment – is always based upon the observations of altered function (e.g. pain, vomiting, weakness) and *precedes* the demonstration and understanding of the causes and structural pathology (if any) of the disease. In fact, it is in the very act of developing a clinical syndrome – the correlating of several signs and symptoms into a single conceptual entity – that we begin to think of and search for a unitary underlying principle.

It is precisely in altered function and sensation rather than altered structure (e.g. chest pain and shortness of breath rather than occlusion of coronary arteries; sugar in the urine rather than some possible submicroscopic or biochemical abnormality within a pancreatic cell) that disease first makes itself known. Once altered function is acknowledged as a criterion for the presence of disease, and the obsolete nature of Szasz's criterion of histopathology is recognized, the way is open to consider what the functions of the brain might be with regard to psychiatric illnesses. From this intermediate step, one can proceed to consider whether logical thinking, language acquisition, social behaviours and emotional regulation are functions of the brain as much as regulation of breathing, coordination of eye–hand movements and body temperature regulation.

There can be no question that abnormalities of physical functioning can be universally recognized. The single stumbling block to transferring this generalization to the psychiatric domain is that the judgement about what constitutes abnormal psychological functioning appears more personally subjective or culturally determined and relies to a larger extent upon the report of the patient. This latter difficulty is itself merely relative, since we are equally dependent upon the report of the patient for evidence of physical dysfunction such as pain, diminished sensation, poor memory, etc. But in general it can be acknowledged that there are profound conceptual and practical difficulties in evaluating what is normal and abnormal in terms of logical thinking, emotional regulation and social behaviour. Behaviour cannot be evaluated out of its physiological, adaptive and social context. Behaviours initially considered pathological would take on a different significance if one discovered the person was play-acting or engaging in some culturally sanctioned ritual. In view of this, are not psychological functions too culture-bound, as well as too much a product of local environment and personal upbringing, for there to be general standards by which to distinguish normal from deviant thinking? If someone does not think as I do, or cries or laughs when I would not, does this mean abnormality and mental illness, and on whose part?

There is a pragmatic answer, which is that whereas minor deviations from 'normality' may be of dubious significance, there is little question for most people in all societies about the significance of severe deviations. If a woman 5 feet 5 inches tall prefers to weigh 92 pounds we might consider this to be a little on the slender side, but as her weight begins to move down to 65 pounds, we ought to become alarmed and insist that this is abnormal, no matter what her own body image purports to be. Similarly, persons can display all sorts of idiosyncrasies in language before we might consider it abnormal, but when their language becomes gibberish and incomprehensible we can properly consider it pathological. There are no absolute standards, just as there are very few in the rest of medicine. One cannot simply take refuge in statistics, considering all conditions that deviate more than two standard deviations from the norm as pathological (although in a statistical sense they are abnormal). In certain parts of the world it may be the norm to have dental caries or to be infested with intestinal parasites, but we would not consider these conditions a state of health. It is not possible to avoid relativistic standards, in which decisions near the mean remain somewhat arbitrary (and therefore call for caution in decision-making) whilst decisions at the extremes are usually so obvious as hardly to require the opinions of professionals. The critical questions remain as to how to apply relativistic standards in the evaluation of deviant social behaviours in the context of health and sickness.

Psychiatric illness in the perspective of evolutionary biology

A model drawn from evolutionary biology must be added to our medical model at this point, but it is not without its own set of problems. The problems in general arise from the difficulty of introducing the concept of 'purpose' and functional adaptation into considerations of health and disease. Nevertheless, unless one wishes to abandon the entire set of Darwinian hypotheses regarding evolution, the concept cannot be avoided. The notion of purpose must be differentiated from an Aristotelian notion of teleology, yet it is clear that both arise from the same observations of how well-suited organisms are to their specific environments. The human brain did not evolve in order that people might develop language and live in a society. Other evolutionary pathways for communication and social organization were certainly possible with a different brain structure – as can be seen in insect societies. But we can say that the particular type of organization of man's brain made possible, and probably accompanied, man's particular development of language and social organizations. Just as it is the kidney's function to remove certain nitrogenous wastes, to assist in maintaining the proper pH and electrolyte balance in the blood, and to assist in blood pressure regulation, so it is among the brain's many functions to adapt man to his social and cultural environment. As Jerison stated,[20]

The work of the brain might be described as creating a real world, through the development of concepts of space, time, and objects. Reality is, thus, a creation of the brain, a model of a possible world that makes sense of the mass of information that reaches us through our various sensory (including motor feedback) systems . . . The peculiarly human relevance of this analysis is for our understanding of the meaning of intelligence as a biological phenomenon. This point of view would consider biologic intelligence as a measure of the quality of the real worlds created by the nervous systems of different species.

There is much mystery about how the brain works, but it is not itself a mysterious organ: it is merely an expanded sensory–motor integration centre of the nervous system placed near the organs of special sense (hearing, vision, smell, taste). And it has developed through evolutionary processes some remarkable functions and some reciprocally remarkable problems. It is hard to conceive of a biological function that cannot somehow go wrong; it is also more likely that a complex system will go wrong in more complicated ways than a simple system.

It seems fairly safe to assert, then, that from an evolutionary point of view one of the major functions of the expanded neocortex of the human brain is language development and acquisition, and that this may be accomplished well or less well. There are many neurological syndromes in which failure of language to develop, or loss of previously acquired language function, as in a stroke in Broca's area, are well documented. There are also several psychiatric syndromes, most notably certain forms of schizophrenia, in which there is well-documented loss of previously acquired language function to a level of idiosyncratic incomprehensibility. No area of gross pathology in such cases comparable to an infarct in Broca's area has yet been discovered. None may be found, although recent work on brain scans of schizophrenics suggests hemispheric asymmetry beyond the bounds of normal variability. But it is nineteenth-century thinking to look only for gross structural defects. It is more likely that abnormalities at a biochemical level (neurotransmitters, receptor sites, and relationships between these) will be discovered in some schizophrenics, but perhaps not all.[21] This is the point our present technology has reached, and it promises in the near future to provide certain answers at certain levels, just as the discovery of a spirochaete as the aetiological agent in syphilis provided certain answers at the turn of the century.

Similarly, there probably are some anatomically localizable areas in the hypo-thalamus that are involved in regulation of mood – by which we mean the maintenance of mood cycles as well as the dampening of environmentally induced changes of mood within certain limits. It is likely that some persons with manic-depressive illness, with extremes of mood high and low, have a disturbance in the functioning of the mood-regulating centre in the hypothalamus.[22] Although this is still hypothetical, there is considerable evidence to support such a hypothesis. Again we can postulate that, from an evolutionary perspective, one function of the brain is to regulate mood, and that a disturbance in this function, which appears to run in families, can properly be called a disease.

There is a problem here to which we have alluded before. This relates to the differences between cultures in deciding what the true (evolutionarily 'desirable') function should be. Is it to be assumed that syllogistic or scientific thinking represents the pinnacle of evolutionary development, and that other types of thinking are dysfunctional, and therefore disturbed, in so far as they differ from syllogistic thinking? And are emotional control and moderation the most adaptive, and therefore healthiest forms of emotional regulation, so that departures from this ideal represent degrees of maladaption and ill-health?

Human beings are social creatures who transmit culture from generation to generation via symbolic communications. Those persons whose characteristic patterns of thought and behaviour are transformed in a manner that renders them unable to communicate, or to maintain the emotional control needed for their peace of mind and safety and for sustaining the interpersonal relationships and social endeavours on which their survival as independent individuals depends can usually be said to have an illness. There are easily imagined examples of situations in which this notion cannot be sustained; these usually involve a radically changed or unusual environment, such as prison, a concentration camp, a lifeboat adrift at sea, conditions of warfare and famine, a governmental reign of terror. Under such unusual circumstances persons may act on principle or out of terror and disorganization in ways that threaten their individual survival or go against the norms of their group. Such behaviour may not indicate mental illness or a failure in the brain's adaptive capability. But such exceptional circumstances do not weaken the general thesis that man's brain has evolved simultaneously with man's social structures and that illness must be viewed in terms of failures of man's functional adaptation. Fabrega has commented on this:[23] 'With regard to the matter of deviation, it seems that the values of the variables that are involved usually deviate both from norms created by the individual's past performance (personal norms) and from norms set by the relevant subgroup to which the person belongs (group norms) . . . From this perspective, the diseases of a people are literally cultural categories.' In essence, adaptive social behaviour is as legitimate and recognizable a product of human evolution as are pulmonary function or bipedal locomotion. Gross disturbances of any of these functions are easy to detect; subtle disturbances are not.

We have seen that a persistent problem in all medical models, but especially a model designed for psychiatry, is how to determine the boundary between normality and abnormality, and what action to take with regard to those individuals who approach this boundary. Two partial answers have been offered so far. First, the boundary is not a line at all, but a vaguely defined band in which individuals have characteristics which depart more or less from normality and approach abnormality. The second is that a perspective derived from evolutionary biology gives us a yardstick with which to evaluate higher brain function, using language and other social abilities. The use of this model is most powerful when considering the major mental illnesses: the schizophrenic and manic-depressive diseases, the 'organic' conditions, and perhaps obsessive-compulsive and other severe neurotic conditions. The greatest difficulties remain over whether and where to place in a health–illness continuum most neurotic disorders, abnormal personalities, and people who have 'problems of living'.

There are two tempting, diametrically opposed solutions to these problems, neither of which is satisfactory. The first is to give in to Szasz's attack, agree with him that the sole criterion of disease is an anatomical or physiological abnormality, and jettison the neuroses, personality disorders and life-stress responses in an attempt to salvage those conditions – such as schizophrenia and manic-depressive disorders – whose biochemical basis is being elucidated at present. Such a manoeuvre would invalidate Szasz's argument regarding civil commitment and the insanity plea in so far as it rests upon his assertion that mental disorders such as schizophrenia do not and cannot have any physical cause. But it would abandon a large number of persons suffering from a variety of disabling conditions such as obsessive-compulsive neurosis, anorexia nervosa and many forms of depression to the harsh moral judgement of fakery, laziness and moral turpitude which is passed when such disorders are isolated from medical considerations. Such a narrowing down of the medical concern for human misery is not justified either by our social values or by our understanding of the complexity of human health and illness.

The second solution is to take the broadest interpretation of the biopsychosocial model and define *all* conditions of distress as illness. This position holds that all determinations of what constitutes illness are cultural decisions. It also holds that since problems of living are contributory factors in the development and maintenance of illnesses, they are therefore forms of illness themselves. However, this very vagueness leads to failures in discrimination between serious and trivial conditions. In addition it fails to help clarify the conditions to which special social and ethical consideration ought to be given, such as eligibility for health care payments and excuse for criminal behaviours. Toulmin has stated this dilemma as follows:[24]

whether the particular individual in any specific situation is indeed a genuine 'patient' to whom something untoward has 'happened' of a kind that takes his case entirely out of the moral sphere – or whether he remains in significant respects an 'agent' who can be, and likely *wants* to be, 'accountable' for conduct which others see as pathological.

The first proposed solution is too restrictive, the second too broad; both pretend to an ease of identifying who has and has not an illness, who is and is not a patient. In our culture psychiatry must grapple not only with the problems raised by the more severe conditions such as schizophrenia and manic-depressive illness, but with problems raised by the common and more ambiguous conditions that make up human life as we know it: neuroses, character quirks, self-destructiveness and aggressiveness, problems in everyday living, anxieties and suspiciousness, high and low intelligence, impulse disorders, and just plain stubbornness. Methods must be developed which can distinguish between these different conditions.

The problem of 'caseness'

The psychiatric profession is aware that it must take scrupulous care to avoid overestimating the scope of the knowledge it possesses and the hypotheses it can formulate. There is already evidence that in common clinical practice psychiatrists are dealing with forms of suffering far removed from the ordinary vicissitudes that are inescapable in the life of individuals of full human stature.

It is well understood that the problems found in certain forms of neuroses and related conditions of human suffering are not easy to differentiate sharply from everyday distress and tribulation. The need to avert the danger of medicalizing social problems is clearly articulated by psychiatrists in many parts of the world.

All modern work on 'caseness' is concerned to discover a criterion of demarcation between ordinary adversity and illness. The evidence that has come to light has shown on the whole that psychiatrists are dealing with forms of suffering which it is humane, sensible, realistic and effective to treat as illness. Bebbington and Tennant's studies have demonstrated that 'most disorders seen in the community are essentially transient distress reactions which are very different in nature from classical depressive illness', and that even the conditions which resemble depressions are much less severe than those which bring people to psychiatrists.[25] While this might appear self-evident, it needed to be demonstrated by a survey that the persons going to psychiatric clinics *differ* from those with the milder type of disorder one discovers in the community. There are of course people in the community in distress. But although there is some overlap, these are generally not the people who attend psychiatric clinics and hospitals. The charge, or the worry, that patients who go to psychiatrists have the common mild problems of living is once again contradicted by the evidence. Psychiatric concern begins when distress goes beyond the ordinary problems both in severity and in duration. And this is a pattern that has stood the test of time.

Throughout this book we have used the terms 'illness' and 'disease' interchangeably, ignoring the distinction posited mainly by sociologists that illnesses are what you think you have and diseases are what you really have.[26] This distinction may be valuable in some contexts, including the practical one of deciding whether or not a person should have surgery. However, in the many cases in which a specific cause or diagnosis cannot be determined, it has been the humane and useful course to assume that the person is ill. Disease models can only be applied in the light of available knowledge and evidence; in this sense many illnesses, including psychiatric ones, appear homologous with the concepts of maladies of unknown cause of a hundred years ago. The decision to consider these as diseases promoted research and the development of methods of diagnosis and treatment for these conditions.

If a person appears unwell and is forced out of his usual pattern of daily life, then it would not be justified to withhold medical care where a specific diagnosis cannot be made or because not all the criteria for disease can be met. It would equally be unjustified to withhold a designation of illness if the person felt well but was discovered to have occult cancer, the early stages of diabetes or hypertension, or a condition such as a frontal lobe tumour or mild mania in which the person will deny the illness and refuse treatment. The denial of illness does not refute the presence of disease.

The boundaries of disease must be flexible. In research one defines the boundaries rigidly; all criteria must be met. In clinical practice one cannot exclude patients because they do not meet all criteria. In fact, throughout history, doctors have been called upon to practise in areas having nothing to do with disease. For example, pregnancy is a state of health, not illness. Yet the inclusion of pregnancy within the domain of medicine has changed the whole situation of childbirth. Only a century ago pregnancy and delivery were very dangerous; labour was considered the most dangerous time in a woman's life. Another example is the area of birth control. This is certainly not a matter of disease, but its complexities are best handled by physicians. Yet despite these examples, medicine has traditionally been concerned not to cross the line into social and political areas.

Are neuroses and character disorders illnesses?

With all these considerations as background, how shall psychiatry legitimately encompass neuroses, personality disorders and severe stress reactions within its domain?

There has been a curious reversal in the thinking and debating about the nature of mental illness during the past few decades. Thirty years ago the dominant psychiatric view was that psychiatric illnesses, even the severe schizophrenic and manic-depressive psychoses, were caused by psychological factors. It was believed that these factors mainly involved early life experiences, such as the basic support and affirmation the child received in passing through the fundamental developmental tasks of a particular culture (bonding, weaning, toilet training, language acquisition, separation from parents, tolerance of frustration). The development of schizophrenia or manic-depressive psychosis in adolescence or early adulthood was attributed to some deficiency of nurture during the first several years of life. There was recognition that in some cases hereditary or constitutional factors might have some importance, but in general this view (and its evidence) was ignored, explained away or even ridiculed. It was regarded by post-Freudians as self-evident and well documented that adverse circumstances, conflict-laden or traumatic at an early age, led to severe emotional problems and mental illnesses.

The 'biological' psychiatrists were in the minority, for after one hundred years of investigation they had come upon no evidence linking either schizophrenia or manic-depressive illness to abnormal structure or function of the central nervous system (assuming one did not consider abnormal behaviour as itself being or reflecting an abnormal function of the central nervous system). The extent of their findings was the general impression that whatever physical or biochemical variable was measured (e.g. serum electrolytes, electroencephalograms, blood pressure), the schizophrenics showed greater variability than a control population.[27] And even this finding might have been the result of chronic illness and hospitalization rather than a biological marker or possible cause of the schizophrenia.

Physical causes of mental illnesses resembling schizophrenia had of course been found, the most famous one being the early stages of central nervous system syphilis; others were amphetamine abuse, pellagra (vitamin B deficiency), some sequelae of chronic alcoholism, occasional brain tumours, and temporal lobe epilepsy. But once these conditions were identified and removed from consideration, a large core group of chronic schizophrenics remained for whom there could be found no organic pathology which might conceivably lead to such a mental and behavioural condition. In addition, it seemed inconceivable that something as biologically gross as a brain tumour or a particular abnormal metabolic pathway could produce the varied and subtle symbolic and linguistic disturbances that are found in schizophrenia.

However, this flirtation with the view that mental illnesses have primarily psychological causes – rising with the development of Freudian psychology and covering at most the period 1900–1970 – is only a brief interlude when seen in historical context. Prior to Freudian thought the dominant European view regarding mental illnesses was that they were organic diseases, often reflecting hereditary forms of nervous system inferiority and degeneration. As G. S. Rousseau has written:

Anatomy and physiology would seem to have been the two shaping forces in the history of psychology. All Western theories of the mind, no matter how primitive, ultimately owe their origin and subsequent development to these two domains, although there are moments when political circumstances (e.g. France 1789–98) are as influential. The history of European psychology can be viewed, to echo Whitehead on Plato, as a footnote on the history of this relation between anatomy and physiology, not merely of the one considered in isolation from the other. While religious and secular concepts also shape psychology, they have not done so to a degree that can compare with the role of anatomy and physiology.[28]

During the 1960s, and certainly by 1970 in the USA, the biological model of mental illnesses had reasserted its dominance, as the power and attractiveness of Freudian psychology declined. In the United Kingdom and western Europe the biological model had never lost its dominant position. The reasons for these dramatic shifts must be many, including both socio-political and medical-scientific factors. Freudian psychology has lost its dominant position in psychiatry (perhaps not in the arts, literature and zeitgeist) for the same reasons as other bodies of theory and data are superseded and partially incorporated in all sciences: the theory is no longer as fruitful as its early promise implied, the hypotheses either could not be tested or were tested and found wanting, and other theories were developed with more fruitful hypotheses, more success in predicting and bringing about change, and seeming better to fit the perceived nature of the world.

However, the antipsychiatry writers such as Szasz, Sarbin and Scheff, and the social labelling theorists, developed their arguments from the model dominant in the 1950s and 1960s.[29] This led them to the conclusion that, as mental illnesses do not reflect demonstrable underlying brain pathology or dysfunction, they are not diseases but deviant social behaviours. The problem is that as the model, and the evidence generated by it, has changed to a broader biological one that also encompasses psychosocial factors, the antipsychiatry writers have been stranded with an obsolete model and an untenable theory. They have merely camouflaged their absence of evidence with more strident arguments.

We are not advocating a reductionist position with regard to the relationship between neural events and mental events.[30] Acknowledgement that the evidence at present points to a major aetiological role for altered brain chemistry and ultrastructure in the development of schizophrenia and manic-depressive illness does *not* imply that there is any understanding at all of *how* altered neurophysiology translates into aberrant thinking. For example, a fair amount is known about the neurophysiology, neurochemistry and endocrinology of aggression in animals and humans.[31] However, knowledge of the pathways of aggression does not enable us to equate the mental state that accompanies or predisposes to aggressiveness with the neurophysiological state itself. Aggression is not a brain state, even if we can specify and measure the physiological configuration of the brain of a person who is being aggressive. Reductionism would equate the two.

Yet we cannot ignore the brain state underlying aggressive behaviour. Suppose that a particular epileptic focus in the temporal lobe led, as far as we could tell, to the development of aggressive behaviour not during a seizure but at other 'ordinary' times, that is, the person over the years slowly but noticeably developed a more aggressive personality. Should we ignore the correlation, and possible causal relationship, between temporal lobe epilepsy and aggressiveness?[32] Or should we consider aggressiveness in this person as a symptom of an organic illness?

Let us consider a situation nearer to normality. Suppose that an aggressive person has a non-specific abnormal brain wave (EEG) pattern. It is not the pattern for epilepsy or any other known condition; it just is abnormal, with an excess of slow activity at too high a voltage when compared with the norms for adults of that age, sex and state of health. Should we attribute some of the aggressiveness, or perhaps some of the inability to tolerate frustration, to the abnormal wave pattern and whatever it indicates as abnormal about the functioning of this particular brain? Suppose we learned that this person had been born after a prolonged labour in which the fetal heartbeat was weak, that the immediate post-natal period was marked by sluggish respiratory response, bluish colouring and poor muscle tone, and that the early developmental landmarks (rolling over, sitting, standing, crawling) came rather late. We may learn also that the aggressive person was physically abused as a child. Is the abuse less of a real event, less of an influence on development than an episode of perinatal anoxia or measles encephalitis which may leave tangible scarring or testable malfunctions? We may have no particular explanation for the aggressiveness. In which circumstances should we call it disease and which not? Should we call aggressiveness plus an abnormal brain wave pattern 'disease' and without an abnormal brain wave pattern a 'normal variant'? But we know that there is no absolutely valid standardization for 'normal' brain wave patterns and that the EEG, picking up the electrical pattern of brain activity in millivolts through skin, scalp, fascia, muscle, skull bone, meninges and cerebrospinal fluid, yields only a very crude approximation of what the brain is actually doing, and even this over the convexity of the brain that represents only a part of the entire cortex. Should we pin our entire decision regarding the presence or absence of disease on this very limited and imprecise diagnostic technique? And is an abnormal brain wave pattern a so much more compelling explanation of agressiveness than a history of repeated childhood beatings that the former represents (or confirms) disease but not the latter?

Margolis has commented: 'The trouble with deciding the medical legitimacy of the concept of mental illness . . . has always been the same, namely, that there are too many analogies and disanalogies between somatic medicine and the variety of disciplines that have centered on alleged mental disorders to decide the matter trimly.'[33] The antipsychiatry writers assert that the classificatory scheme they prefer and the definition of disease they use are accurate reflections of nature rather than pragmatic conventions. It is as though their classificatory scheme carved nature at its joints – assuming that nature has joints or discontinuities – and that they have discovered these. But there are no strong arguments for either of these assumptions. We have a diagnostic system that divides diseases into discrete categories because we find it easier to think and work this way, not because it is a more 'accurate' representation of how things are in nature. Thus we designate a diastolic blood pressure above 90 mm mercury as hypertension (meaning that we will probably attempt to lower any blood pressure above that level) and we similarly designate a fasting blood sugar level above 120 mg/100 ml as hyperglycaemic and probably indicative of diabetes. But these are clearly working conventions for our own convenience; there is no external validation that pressures above 90 mm mercury *really* are hypertensive. The case is similar for mental retardation, obesity, thyroid functioning, joint disease and coronary insufficiency. Although the end points are easy to determine, it remains unclear where health shades into illness at the near end of the spectrum.

In essence, some critics of psychiatry assume a black–white dichotomy and therefore assert that everything is either one thing or the other, that there are no shades of grey, no conditions or examples which do not fit into the either–or model of the universe. However, since this line of reasoning goes against common sense and one's own experience, there are good reasons for rejecting their assertions and for adopting models that approximate more closely the world as we know it. In this world, tones of black shade imperceptibly into grey and grey into white. Neat boundaries are hard to find.

The way the world is represented is not only a simple matter of style or preference: it is also a matter of evidence. The classification must be workable for the purposes intended – useful now and promising advances in the future. But it is not on account of any alleged failure in these respects that Szasz objects to the inclusion of mental illness within the schema of disease. His objection is rather that such a concept of disease is *incorrect*, that it does not accurately reflect nature. And this, as we have seen, completely misunderstands the nature of classification, and, possibly, the nature of nature.

Perhaps it is best that we acknowledge at the outset that we have no satisfactory answers regarding the neuroses and character disorders. It is clear that some of these conditions are learned; they appear to evolve to a considerable extent from life experiences. Most cases have little somatic basis that could be differentiated from normal somatic and neurophysiological functioning. It is equally clear that more and more evidence is being discovered which points toward an inherited basis for many aspects of temperament and personality which we formerly believed had come about strictly as a result of life experiences. Studies of identical twins separated at birth have revealed startling similarities in temperament and taste that appear to defy the possibility of coincidence. Traits such as shyness, characteristics such as anxiety-proneness, and preferences toward criminal addictive behaviours appear to occur on a partially genetic basis.[34] It is not clear yet how to integrate these findings with our traditional beliefs that these personality features are the result of social learning.

The volitional disorders

There is in medicine a group of disorders often referred to as 'volitional' disorders. The term is applied to self-destructive behaviours which people seem to perform voluntarily and which, if not representing an illness in themselves, certainly tend to cause serious medical problems if the behaviours are not interrupted. Of course the term 'volitional' rests on a particular assumption that glosses over a major philosophical quandary: to what extent are seemingly volitional acts actually volitional and to what extent are they 'determined' by a combination of psychodynamic, behavioural and neurophysiological antecedents? This is the venerable free will/ determinism problem which is not here in question. The present use of the concept of 'volitional disorders' presupposes that there *is* a problem of intentionality only in order to investigate the antecedents of actions and behaviours in such conditions, should we call them 'free' or 'unfree'.

Examples of volitional disorders which in general are regarded by physicians as proper to medicine are: anorexia and bulimia nervosa, wrist-cutting and overdosing with pills, obesity, and alcohol and drug abuse. In all these cases investigators have attempted – with some success – to demonstrate that there are in fact biochemical or neurophysiological differences between groups exhibiting these disorders and normal groups. Whether these differences really operate as causal factors of self-destructive behaviour is at present open to conjecture. In the eyes of some, such evidence tends to legitimate the organic aspect of these disorders. But it is not clear why knowledge of some of the physiological antecedents, rather than of the psychological and experiential antecedents of behaviour should provide a better justification that a disorder is 'less volitional' and therefore more properly medical.

To carry the argument further, there are other types of behaviour which appear unrelated to illness, yet the continuous performance of these behaviours might make these persons as much a subject of medical care as those with bulimia, anorexia or alcoholism. Consider cigarette smoking and refusal to take exercise. Do not these behaviours place the person at greater risk in almost all major categories of disease? Consider other risk-taking behaviours, such as engaging in sexual perversions with violent strangers. Let us examine such a situation a little more closely.

A 27-year-old man requested hospitalization for his emotional problems. He narrated a history of increasingly dangerous masochistic behaviour which he felt powerless to stop. He would go to homosexual bars or pick up strangers on the street. His request in these liaisons was that he be tied up prior to sexual activity. His choice of partners veered toward psychopathic characters, and he had in the past been burned with cigarettes, cut with razors, and beaten into unconsciousness. He would vow after these occasions never to do it again, but within a few weeks or so would start going to the same bars, or drive to a new town where he was not known and pick up a stranger. He stated that he felt compelled to do this despite (or because of) his awareness of the risks. He narrated a history of parental abuse when he was a child. About one year after this hospitalization, this man was tied up and brutally murdered in his apartment, with evidence of several hours of mutilation and torture prior to his death.

We are dealing here with seemingly compulsive behaviour. There is a repetitive pattern of conduct which has potentially serious consequences for his health, and which had already led to burns, razor cuts and head injury. And the man feels powerless to stop. The nature of the aetiology is not clear, nor is it particularly logical to say that we would categorise this as a medical problem if there were a hormonal imbalance and not if there were only psychological determinants. The person suffers from a specific pattern of behaviour which *he* sees as abnormal, and he is asking for help. Except for the absence of cellular pathology, this situation would appear to meet the requirements for disease status. Might we not describe epilepsy in similar terms? It is important that concerns about the moral aspect of the symptomatic behaviour should not interfere with the judgement as to whether or not this is illness and whether it is worthy of medical attention. Suppose the patient seeking help was a 'house-proud' housewife, whose obsessive preoccupations with germs and compulsive house-cleaning led to antagonism and separation from her husband, alienation from her children, inability to leave the house because it was never clean enough, and a peptic ulcer. Would our considerations be any different?

There does appear to be a spectrum of human behaviours along which we can locate conditions that resemble medical conditions to a greater or lesser degree. Where on this spectrum we place any particular individual or any particular condition depends not just on the inherent features of the person or condition; rather it represents a complex social judgement based upon the total cultural approach to conditions of infirmity and deviance.

Throughout this book we have spoken mainly about schizophrenia and manic-depressive illness, and about probable brain mechanisms underlying both normal and abnormal behaviours. We have said very little about neuroses and character disorder. This is because the continuity of psychiatric illnesses within the larger domain of medical illnesses is most easily, as well as most importantly, demonstrated in the cases of schizophrenia and manic-depressive illness. Even in these cases, however, it has been essential to demonstrate that the continuity goes both ways. At one extreme each of these conditions has already been shown to be associated with organic lesions or diseases in a proportion of cases. At the other extreme some problems of demarcation arise from the range of the norm in behaviour. As we have commented earlier, modern science has achieved its remarkable progress by isolating smaller and smaller bits of large systems in order to analyse these bits in greater detail. The systems analysed do not have to be exclusively physiological ones. It is perfectly legitimate, and even necessary, to carry out analysis at the psychological and sociological levels of human functioning. This division of labour is not entirely artificial. Each level of description and investigation has its own methods and integrity, and a loose correlation between the levels can be achieved. It is not that one level of analysis is more correct or more profound than another.

At present the neuroses and character disorders are most usefully examined at the behavioural and introspective levels. The degree to which specific brain mechanisms will be discovered underlying neurotic and characterological disorders, and which of these mechanisms will be considered abnormal, remains for the future to discover. These expected discoveries will not invalidate the basic achievements of Freudian psychology. These achievements include the hypothesis of the basic lawfulness of human thought and behaviour at the psychological level, and the assertion that psychological disturbances have psychological causes, not just physical ones.

Our use of dualistic language, such as in distinguishing psychological and physical causes, is based upon the limitations inherent in the assumptions of our language and refers to levels of analysis, not to a separation of mind and body. It was Freud himself who emphasized the continuity between normal and disturbed behaviour, between everyday slips and forgetfulness and the more profound thought and memory disturbances. Although one can say that the poets and playwrights of all eras have understood that the 'child is father of the man' it was not until the twentieth century that the historical dimension, the need to look before and after in order to study and understand human behaviour, was spelled out within a scientific framework. Bruner has commented on this:[35]

it is our heritage from Freud that the all-or-none distinction between mental illness and mental health has been replaced by a more humane conception of the continuities of these states. The view that neurosis is a severe reaction to human trouble is as revolutionary in its implications for social practice as it is daring in formulation.

The concept of a continuity between health and illness at both the psychological and physiological levels has specific implications for social practice. These will be discussed in the next chapter.

We cannot prove that neuroses and personality disorders are illnesses, because this is not the sort of issue that is amenable to proof. We have to compare the ways in which they resemble other conditions which are considered illnesses in our society; we also have to consider the totality of consequences for the person and those about him if the condition is considered an illness, and the alternative consequences if it is considered not to be an illness. To place these disorders within the medical model is to make a judgement about the weight of the available evidence and a forecast of the likely outcome of future research.[36] It also makes medical care properly available to persons incapacitated with such conditions. The alternative, according to Szasz's recommendations, is to place schizophrenics and neurotics in the categories of criminals, spongers, charlatans and inadequates, and to deny them access to medical care. In view of the suffering and reduced level of functioning of most persons with neurotic and personality disorders, there is more than ample justification for placing these conditions within a medical model of illness.

6 Social, ethical and philosophical aspects of involuntary hospitalization and the insanity defence

The previous chapters have dealt with scientific hypotheses and facts, and with empirical statements which, in principle, could either be confirmed or refuted by observation and experimentation. The present chapter is concerned primarily with values, not facts.[1] Issues of fact are fairly clear in terms of what is known, what is not known, and what evidence there is for what we hypothesize but do not yet know. Issues of value are never clear or beyond dispute. This is especially true if the factual basis upon which we argue our values has not been sufficiently clarified in previous critical discussions of the problem.

Our facts, as best we know them, may indicate that a mentally ill person with a thought-disorganized type of schizophrenia will not be able to earn a living or even look after himself without assistance. We may also know that the incoherence of thought will improve appreciably if the person takes antipsychotic medication, but that there is a possibility the person will develop side-effects of the medication (tremors, stiffness and involuntary movements) and that in a minority these may be lasting. These are the facts and probabilities. It is a question of values whether society wishes to support such unfortunate persons, and whether society will insist on hospitalizing persons who appear unable to care for themselves to such a degree that they may starve or commit suicide. It is a question of values whether society should insist that such persons take medication whether they want to or not. To answer these questions it must first be decided in particular whether the benefits of medication outweigh the risks of side-effects, in general whether the benefits of a paternalistic social policy outweigh the risks of ever-broader governmental intrusion into personal choice and liberty, and whether we believe that mentally ill persons are the casualties of capitalist societies and whether we wish to use these mentally ill persons as sacrificial shock troops in a class struggle.

Thus we ask of science questions relating to whether something *can* be done and, if so, how, and with what consequences. We ask of values whether something *ought* to be done, in view of the process itself, the knowledge we possess, and the consequences. Although issues of values cannot be resolved by issues of facts, they often rely heavily on an accurate appraisal of facts, and on the ability to distinguish between facts, conjectures and opinions.

There are two separate but interrelated topics to be discussed, and there is considerable controversy about both.

82

1   Does society have the right, and perhaps obligation, to impose care and treatment for the incapacitated mentally ill, even against their wishes?

2   Should persons with mental illness be held responsible for their criminal behaviours?

There are assumptions involved in the very framing of these questions and these must be made explicit, for they determine the categories and range within which we can seek answers. In a general sense there is the assumption that questions about such complex phenomena can even be framed and answered. The act of asking a question and having the question accepted as legitimate implies that it can be answered in its present form. This deceptively simple concession often leads to problems as the argument unfolds, when it may appear that the shape of the question involved one in a logical or empirical trap. In the present field there is a temptation to accept as legitimate a question so framed as to require a yes/no answer. This often does great injustice to the richness of the subject matter.

We are mainly concerned with matters of degree, of 'more or less' rather than 'present or absent'. This shows up most clearly in our selection of terms. What do we mean by 'care and treatment'? Do we mean custodial care, actively pursued milieu care, or aggressive pharmacological and electroconvulsive treatments? What do we mean by 'incapacitated'? How incapacitated does a mentally ill person have to be: Unable to work? Unable to obtain shelter from the rain or heat? Unable to ignore the persistent hallucinatory voice that tells him to kill himself? What do we mean by 'mental illness'? Do we include only persons who are incoherent, or persons who are paranoid, and if so, how paranoid? Are there degrees of paranoia, and how would we measure this? Do we include mania or depression? Do we include kleptomania and passive–aggressive personality? For 'responsible', do we mean in a limited degree or fully responsible? How can we ever satisfactorily infer that a person could not have done otherwise?

Involuntary commitment based on dangerousness to self

It is essential at the outset to make explicit that the majority of patients treated in mental hospitals and clinics are there voluntarily. This is true even of psychotic, severely depressed and suicidal patients, who receive care within the context of the ordinary doctor–patient relationship based upon trust and confidence. It is only a small minority of patients who are involuntarily committed to hospital. Since these patients represent an area of controversy in psychiatry, they will be the focus of the following two sections.

The civil commitment statutes of most jurisdictions recognize three conditions resulting from mental illnesses which justify involuntary commitment (and in some cases and some jurisdictions, involuntary treatment).[2] These are dangerousness to self, dangerousness to others, and inability to care for one's basic needs or to avoid dangerous exploitation. Mental illness in the absence of these conditions is not grounds for civil commitment. Since most people agree that civil commitment, i.e. involuntary incarceration of a person who has not committed a crime, and involuntary treatment (based upon what others believe is best for a person) represent *massive* infringements of that person's civil liberties and personal integrity, it follows that the factual basis and the ethico-legal justification for such a course must be suitably strong and unambiguous. But issues of probabilities and values can never be without ambiguities. In reality, we are speaking of degrees of severity of mental illness, predictions of dangerousness, and competing ethical systems.

Consider the following five case vignettes, taken from our clinical practices, in which temporary restriction of liberty would appear to be inescapable in the interests of both the patients, their families and society – and life-saving. They represent a cross-section of the types of problems that have to be dealt with by hospitals and emergency rooms. Some cases require immediate decisions by physicians, who fully recognize that the information upon which a decision is based is inevitably incomplete.

Case 1

R. L. is a 32-year-old unemployed shoe salesman. He is married and has two young children. He has had two depressive episodes, the first of which required hospitalization. Following his second depression he became progressively more active and excited to the point of elation. One morning he left his family and began flying from city to city, staying in hotels and eating in restaurants, charging all his expenses to his credit card. While in each city he began purchasing shoe stores, including inventories. The business deals, of course, never went through, because there was no money in the bank to support his down-payments, nor did he have any credit. Each time his family received news of his location they would try to contact him, only to discover that he had already left the hotel and, presumably, the city. He had charged well over $5000 in airfares and daily expenses before his family caught up with him. He insisted that he was a millionaire and was going to corner the retail shoe business of the nation.

Case 2

G. B. is a 28-year-old, single physiotherapist. She has a six-year history of inflicting injuries upon herself or simulating serious medical problems and then requesting care in emergency rooms where she is unknown. She has used atropine drops in one eye to dilate her pupil and simulate a head injury. This led to an emergency lumbar puncture and several days of hospitalization. She has injected bacteria into her bloodstream, causing septicaemia with chills and high fever. She has splashed sulphuric acid into her eyes. Since she often does not report her own role in the development of these conditions, she usually undergoes extensive, expensive, and sometimes painful and risky diagnostic investigations. On one occasion she flew to another city and injected herself with insulin, thereby causing herself to have a seizure (secondary to hypoglycaemia) at the airport. She has also presented herself in emergency rooms complaining of severe abdominal pain. She has had several abdominal exploratory operations. She has also had several cystoscopies (passing a thin telescope into her bladder) because she added a few drops of blood to her urine specimen.

Case 3

M. V. is a 48-year-old married geologist with three teenage children. He was born in Holland and was captured during the Japanese invasion of Sumatra in World War II. He came to the United States in the 1950s and within a decade discovered that he had progressive kidney failure. He was maintained on kidney dialysis and then became one of the early kidney transplant recipients. About three days after the operation he became delirious for about one week. During this time he thought he was being pursued in the jungles of Sumatra. On several occasions he tried to leap out of his fifth-storey window. Since his medical condition was precarious and required the specialized care of the kidney transplant team, he was kept in restraints in his bed on the surgical ward until his delirium cleared.

Case 4

W. G. is a 34-year-old, divorced assembly-line worker. He has had several periods of depression in the past which did not lead to hospitalization. For several months following his divorce he was noticed by his parents, with whom he lived, and by his friends at work, to be increasingly despondent. He spoke a few times about being better off dead. One morning, instead of going to work, he waited nearby until his parents had both left for work. He returned to the house and drove his car into the garage. He sealed up the window and door cracks with newspapers, connected a long hose, previously purchased and hidden, from the car exhaust to the inside of the car and turned on the engine. He was found unconscious some time later and pulled out of the garage by his foreman, who had become worried when W. G. did not arrive at work. W. G. was hospitalized on an intensive care ward. Upon recovery, he appeared to have considerable memory loss. However, he was still despondent and requested his discharge.

Case 5

A. N. is an 18-year-old schoolgirl. One year ago she became socially
withdrawn and lost interest in her studies. She became preoccupied with
religious questions and spent hours reading the Bible. She reported that
she heard voices calling her a sinner and commanding her to hurt herself.
One day she darted in front of a moving car in response to such a command.
She sustained bruises, but no fractures or internal injuries. She refused to
see a psychiatrist or a counsellor. Her hygiene and grooming began to
deteriorate, and she spent long periods of time staring into space,
occasionally grimacing and frowning. Her parents admitted her to an open
psychiatric ward at the local general hospital. Three days later, A. N. walked
off the ward, took the lift to the fifth floor, and jumped out of a window.
She sustained a broken wrist, shoulder, ribs and pelvis, and a ruptured
spleen. She stated that she jumped because the voice of Satan commanded
her.

In summary, Case 1 depicts a 32-year-old manic man who is grandiose and
travels around the country spending money he does not have. He has put his
impecunious family deeply in debt and shows no sign of slowing down. He may
be charged with fraud. There is no evidence that either he or anyone else is in
imminent physical danger as a result of his behaviour, although it is possible he
may get himself assaulted because of his verbally aggressive behaviour and poor
judgement. His behaviour, however, is recognized by his family as highly abnormal
and out of character. When his family (wife and father) catch up with him, they
ask the court to commit him.

Case 2 is much more problematic, and was included in the series for that reason.
It involves a young woman who is not psychotic but who places herself at
considerable medical risk to pursue a strongly felt need to receive emergency
medical attention. Her family has severed nearly all contact with her, but her
boyfriend wants to have her committed. The patient herself acknowledges that
there is something wrong with her, but does not think hospitalization will help
nor does she wish to be hospitalized.

From the standpoint of Szasz, Sarbin and others, such individuals are liars and
cheats. Such a judgement adopts the rigid, uncompassionate and intimidating
attitude of the most reactionary of physicians of the past. Obviously conscious
falsification on the part of the patients is involved. But the reasons underlying the
behaviours are completely concealed. These cases, in our view, are the most
malignant forms of disorders manifest in hysterical personalities, and they have
a compelling claim on patient, tolerant and imaginative care from physicians.[3] The
dilemma is created by the fact that treatment that is sustained over a long period,
particularly for those patients able to acknowledge their own active participation

in simulation of disease, is rewarded. We have seen individuals of high achievement and long dedication to careers in nursing, medicine and religious orders, among others, restored to their social role. We have also seen others die from their prolonged illnesses.

The question arises whether such individuals should be committed in the manner of suicidal patients. To our knowledge, it is repugnant to psychiatrists to take such action, but it is for society to discuss this issue and express its view regarding what legal action it would like to see to avert the tragic waste of lives.

Case 3 is that of a man who suffers a post-operative delirium and will undoubtedly, if not restrained, either hurt himself directly or interfere with his post-operative recovery and chances of a successful kidney transplant. It is expected that his delirium will clear and that he will not have to be kept restrained indefinitely.

Case 4 describes a man who was seriously depressed and methodically went about his suicide attempt. Does it make a difference in our willingness to commit a suicidally depressed person whether the depression appears to be a response to unfortunate life events or appears to come out of the blue, with no obvious precipitating causes? Can we say that the 'biologically caused' depression is a medical illness and therefore justifies commitment, whereas the 'psychologically caused' depression just demonstrates the person's moral weakness and lack of resilience in giving in to sadness and therefore does not justify commitment?

Case 5 offers an almost classical description of the slow inexorable development of schizophrenia in an adolescent, beginning with social withdrawal, making use of an available cultural pattern (in this case, religiosity) and ending in a frank psychotic state with hallucinations which command self-destructive behaviour. No one appreciated the seriousness of her psychotic absorption in a private religious system unrestrained by moderating influences. When she recovered from the injuries of the fall, she tried to kill herself by leaping off her radiator backwards into her room on her head.

We have presented vignettes of actual case histories, not stylized examples which bleach out the intricate social networks found in life. We have stressed repeatedly throughout this book that the decisions involved are hard, precisely because complexities and uncertainties abound. The manic man is clearly ill to all who know him, but he is infused with a sense of well-being, even euphoria. He does not want to interrupt his cross-country buying spree, and appears oblivious of the expenses he is incurring. We can cite this case as an argument for the evils of credit cards, or take refuge in the possibility that he can declare himself bankrupt and let the hotels, restaurants, shops and airlines absorb the loss. We can even say that his personal liberty is worth more than the five or ten thousand dollars his family may have to borrow to pay his debts. But his manic state is not his normal self; it is a state of illness. It represents a distinct and sudden shift to a style of thinking and behaviour that is alien to his former personality. The choice is to commit him to involuntary hospitalization and treatment with lithium (assuming he refuses to return home and take medication) or to respect his right to be psychotic and perhaps to ruin himself and his family.

Furthermore, most manic patients, after recovery, and their families, express gratitude for the care and protection that has been afforded them and the help that has enabled them to return to their normal social role. Many learn to recognize the early warnings of manic-depressive disease and report to their psychiatrists for help in bringing the disease under control. Complaints, criticism and legal action against psychiatrists for illegal commitment do occur, but are rare in the extreme. Critics of psychiatry might contest such statements and also question the authenticity of the satisfaction and gratitude displayed by manic-depressive patients after treatment. The results of modern methods of treatment in this group of disorders and the effects on patients' lives have been fully documented by psychiatrists. No evidence from critics of psychiatry is on record: only assertions.

An episode of indubitable mania is not a benign condition; it is not one of the slight quirks which the social labelling theorists so lightly refer to as minor deviances. The prognosis for untreated manic-depressive illnesses is one of increasing frequency and severity of recurrences, with briefer intervals of health over the years, or death.[4] It is likely that the acute manic episode of the man described in Case 1 would respond rapidly to antipsychotic and lithium medications, and that future manic and depressive episodes could in most instances be prevented with prophylactic lithium therapy. These are not conjectures, but well-documented and established medical facts. We need to appreciate the effectiveness of treatment and the poor prognosis without treatment in reaching our judgement about the value of commitment.

However, the establishment of the relevant medical facts can only provide the background against which a judicial decision must be made. The judicial decision must take into account the additional facts that diagnostic assessments entail some inaccuracy, that in some persons the risk to themselves of not committing them has been overestimated, and that not all cases improve with medical treatment. The presence of this grey area regarding uncertain diagnosis and uncertain risk of self-injury makes it certain that some persons will be admitted to hospital whose mental illness does not carry a substantial risk of self-injury. Anyone answerable for the life and safety of mentally ill patients and able to make only the imperfect predictions permitted by actuarial and clinical data is bound to err on the side of caution and safety. The penalties for doing otherwise are disproportionately high. But in the presence of these uncertainties, who shall take the risk and assume the responsibility for overestimating or underestimating danger?

The legal tradition of our Western democracies is that, when there is uncertainty, society should bear the risk. But this question is usually framed in cases in which society itself is at risk of harm if the person in question remains free. In cases of illnesses leading to self-injury, the patient is at risk of suicide, serious injury, or family disruption and ruin if he retains his freedom. Society, except indirectly or as regards those immediately concerned, runs little risk from maintaining the self-dangerous person in the community.

The medical viewpoint, in the minority of cases where the degree of immediate risk is uncertain, leans at the present time towards admission on a voluntary basis, or where this is not possible, towards commitment. We consider the risk of incorrect diagnosis in cases of severe mental disturbances to be very small compared with the risk of destruction of life, family, livelihood and career.

The attitudes and policies of society should therefore give due weight to the need to institute psychiatric care at an early stage of illness, to take account of the benefits that patients, their families and the community would derive from such policies. However, the laws relating to mental health in a number of countries have of late given priority to quite other considerations. Alan Stone has described the consequences of the reforms recently introduced in the United States partly under the influence of the civil rights movement.[5] Danger to others rather than severity of illness and need for treatment has become the *main* criterion for civil commitment of psychiatrically ill patients to mental hospital. But the use of the standards and procedures of the criminal law for committing patients to mental hospital has failed in its central objective of protecting the public from dangerous mentally ill patients. It has also ignored society's responsibility to those mentally ill persons who are in danger of hurting themselves either directly through suicidal and other self-destructive behaviours, or indirectly through neglect of themselves and refusal of treatment. This has shown up most clearly in the large number of mentally ill persons who are now, as a result of the policy of deinstitutionalization, living homeless, without medical care, and without protection from predators, in the large cities of the United States[6] and in Italy (as discussed in Chapter 1).

Legal intervention in decisions relating to treatment has led to a lower standard of responsibility to patients as persons. Denied the right to treat patients in the manner demanded by the best available knowledge, psychiatrists are reduced by legal decisions to the role of gaolers. Families have been alienated, psychiatrists driven from the public sector, and a complex bureaucracy has supplanted the clinician in some of his roles.[7] And it is impossible, in situations of crisis or disaster, to determine where responsibility lies. In this state of incoherence of the law, further reforms cannot be far off. In the meantime, lives are placed at risk.

This point is clearly demonstrated in the five cases we have presented. Some of them, such as the delirious kidney transplant patient and the psychotic teenager, appear to be so obviously in need of external safeguards as scarcely to warrant comment. The implications are different for each, in that the delirious man can be expected to recover shortly, as may the manic patient. The teenager may show some improvement with antipsychotic treatment, but it is possible that she will never recover completely and may require intermittent or continuous hospitalization to prevent her from killing herself. The other two cases are more problematic, especially the young woman who presented at emergency rooms with factitious illness, often called Munchausen syndrome. There is a chance that she will accidentally kill or permanently injure herself. She is not psychotic. She does feel compelled to continue her simulations of illnesses, but it is not clear what it means when someone says they cannot stop an action that appears to everyone else to be voluntary.[8] The man who attempted to kill himself with the fumes of a car exhaust has already incurred some brain damage. It remains for the future to discover whether the damage is reversible or permanent, and whether he will try to kill himself again if his depression is not treated effectively.

Establishing guidelines for risk of self-injury

Involuntary commitment, as well as pleading insanity as an excuse for criminal behaviour, is often criticized because the legal definitions of mental illness and insanity are unsatisfactory. As soon as new definitions or new tests for mental illness are proposed, they are roundly attacked and their inevitable weaknesses or circularity ridiculed. Definitions of mental illness use terms such as 'abnormality of mind', 'substantial impairment', 'substantial incapacity', 'defect of reason', and 'not know the nature and quality of an act'. That concepts of illness are difficult to define is sometimes used to argue that no one is mentally ill or that the laws about sanity and insanity are so vague as to be unconstitutional. And if the laws are not clear, neither in many cases are the clinical predictions. It is well known, for example, that psychiatrists and psychologists predict many more suicides than actually occur. However, there is a considerable body of knowledge about the factors correlated with suicide: physical illness, recent losses, schizophrenic and depressive illnesses, previous suicide attempts, family history and lack of support systems.[9]

We are left then with guidelines rather than absolute prescriptions in a variety of very difficult situations. Without intervention, three of the five cases outlined above will probably be dead, one may damage herself, and the manic man will probably destroy his family and social situation, if not himself. If we intervene, we take away freedom of action and impose our will and values.

Szasz's solution that intervention is never justified ignores all the difficulties in these agonizing situations. First of all, it completely ignores the concept of diminished capacity, a concept as real as it is vague. The kidney transplant patient is suffering from a toxic psychosis. He is not oriented to his surroundings and does not appreciate the consequences of climbing out the window. The schizophrenic teenager is responding to hallucinations. Surely in these cases we must intervene.

Second, the amount of hardship and suffering undergone by the family of the mentally ill and suicidal person must be taken into account. To invoke such images risks melodrama, but suicides do leave behind children, spouses and parents who are damaged by such acts. Children and spouses are deprived of the physical presence and financial and emotional support of the suicide. The children especially are left with a legacy of bewilderment, guilt and pain. It is not as though suicide is inevitable, the blind unfolding of one's fate. Most suicides arise out of a specific grouping of unfortunate events and/or a specific episode of illness. If the illness is treated, or the seemingly overwhelming nature of the events is allowed with time to recede into perspective, nearly all would-be suicides can return to reasonably stable and productive lives.

Third, many people who attempt suicide unsuccessfully inflict upon themselves considerable physical damage, creating more intractable social and familial problems and disability than were present before the attempt. There are would-be suicides who have given themselves frontal lobotomies from pistol wounds, shot off their jaws, caused serious neurological impairment and diminished intelligence with carbon monoxide poisoning and insulin overdose, and have permanently paralysed themselves from the neck down by jumping from heights. Shall we say that it serves them right?

There is a value-system that under all circumstances reveres freedom of choice above all other considerations. This appears to be based on the fear that once freedoms can be curtailed for any reason, even to save the life of a person who would surely thank us when recovered, then the erosion of freedoms will follow swiftly and inexorably. Therefore it is better to let a few suicidal people, mentally ill or not, die rather than risk our liberties. But it is not a case of a few suicides. In the United States suicide is the seventh greatest cause of death in all males, and tenth in all females. In 1976 there were 28 800 deaths by suicide there, yielding a rate of 12.5 per 100 000 population. Suicide is the second greatest cause of death (behind accidents) in the United States in males *and* females aged 15–24, and the fourth greatest cause in males and females aged 25–44. The suicide rate increases with age, although its relative standing drops because of the greater increases in death rates from 'natural' causes. The figures are comparable in Great Britain, where suicide is the third greatest cause of death (behind accidents and neoplasms) in males and females (combined figure) aged 15–24, and third (behind neoplasms and circulatory diseases) in males and females aged 25–44. Suicide drops to fifth place for males and females aged 45–54, and to sixth place for those aged 55–64.[10] Most though not all suicides can be attributed to mental illnesses, but the incidence of suicide is probably under-reported, since many deaths recorded as due to accidents and other causes may actually have been suicides.

Szasz exemplifies the libertarian viewpoint's inability to appreciate that complex problems do not admit of simple solutions. He points out that much evil in the world has been done by people who insist upon helping others. This is true. But much evil in this world also results from standing by and not providing help when it ought to be forthcoming. The question is whether we can have confidence that our laws and law courts will strike a reasonable balance between respect for individual liberty and responsibility for preventing mentally ill persons from destroying themselves. The 1959 Mental Health Act of Great Britain was heralded as the most advanced and far-seeing piece of social legislation of this century. It took the care of mental illness out of the courts and leaned entirely on clinical judgement. Psychiatrists, other physicians, and the helping professions were the only ones involved in commitment. This was recognized as making for greater humanity and efficiency in the treatment of mentally ill persons. In Great Britain, since the 1959 Mental Health Act, the great majority of mentally ill persons have been admitted to hospital voluntarily, without involvement of lawyers or courts.

There is admittedly the danger that the zealousness of the helpers might tend to outweigh the caution of the jurists, and that the helpers might ignore – as they have in the past – the high number of false positives (those who would not have hurt themselves) unnecessarily committed to overcrowded institutions and given ineffective treatment. But in the United States in recent years, excessive zeal in the opposite direction has loomed up as the greater danger. Mentally ill persons who could have been successfully cared for by short-term treatment have been denied the protection of civil commitment. There is agitation in Great Britain for legislation on similar lines. This would be a retrograde step. It is our view that at the present time the diagnostic and therapeutic procedures of the major mental illnesses, those which untreated lead to suicide, are so reliably established that a proper balance can be maintained between protection against suicide and protection of liberty.

Involuntary commitment based on dangerousness to others

Involuntary commitment of persons allegedly mentally ill and dangerous to others poses problems similar to those raised by suicidal persons with respect to identification and prediction, but vastly different ethical and social problems. In the case of persons mentally ill and dangerous, the state does not pursue involuntary commitment primarily for the good of the person (although preventing the person from assaulting or murdering someone is most likely in that person's best interest). Rather, the state invokes its police power to protect other citizens from possible harm inflicted by a mentally ill person who has not as yet (in most cases) harmed anyone during *this* episode of mental illness.*

---

*Many qualifying phrases are needed because in fact the mentally ill person may have threatened others, which is a form of harm, or may actually have assaulted others in a manner which did little damage and would not otherwise result in a prison sentence, but which, in combination with the mental illness, appears to foreshadow unacceptable risk of harm to others.

Since the present controversy involves those cases in which no actual assault or battery has occurred, we shall confine our discussion to this class of situations. Thus the mentally ill person is at risk of involuntary commitment and all that such a procedure entails because family and certain other parties (usually professionals such as psychiatrists) predict that he is likely to harm someone else. Adding to the unsatisfactoriness of this situation is the widely quoted inability of psychiatrists to agree on a diagnosis and the even greater inability of psychiatrists (or anyone else for that matter) to predict accurately the future behaviour of others – especially who will and who will not be violent in the future. Furthermore, the concept of 'future' is vague. How far in the future: the next twenty-four hours, the next week, the next month, or the next two years? It is one thing to detain someone for three days if there is sufficient reason to believe that violence is imminent; quite another thing to hold someone for several years because it is predicted that violence will occur sometime in the indefinite future. Finally, there is good evidence that, for a variety of understandable reasons, psychiatrists tend to err on the conservative or safe side (from society's point of view) and overpredict dangerousness, preferring to commit too many, rather than risk future violence from a person for whom they predicted non-violence.

Steadman summarizes the problem from the legal point of view as follows:

Since the use of predictions of dangerousness are really products of the state's rights to protect its citizens, the question arises as to how often the state can be justified in detaining persons as dangerous who would not actually display the predicted behaviour. That is, what is an acceptable false positive rate? That is, of course, a social policy question that frequently parades as a medical question of clinical judgement.[11]

Ennis and Litwack reach the same conclusion:

Human behaviour is difficult to understand, and, at present, impossible to predict. Subject to constitutional limitations, the decision to deprive another human of liberty is not a psychiatric judgement but a social judgement. We shall have to decide how much we value individual freedom; how much we care about privacy and self-determination; how much deviance we can tolerate – or how much suffering. There are no 'experts' to make those decisions for us.[12]

If the facts concerning the risks of violence to society are not clear, then the risk of error of diagnosis or prediction ought not to fall on the person accused; the burden of proof rests with society. These are compelling arguments for cautiousness in the use of involuntary commitment. They are not compelling arguments that commitment is never necessary. There is another side to the debate, another marshalling of both scientific evidence and human suffering which must be added into the balance for each individual determination.

Szasz as usual is unable to find any arguments which might balance out the single *summum bonum* of individual liberty at all costs. His solution is to abolish involuntary commitment completely, except perhaps for a few aggressive paranoids whose threats of violence cannot be ignored. In a remarkable article in *The New Republic*,[13] he comments on recent reports that psychiatrists are being more and more often assaulted, and even murdered, by psychiatric patients. Szasz depicts psychiatrists as finally getting their just and long overdue deserts. He refers to psychiatrists as masters and patients as slaves. He writes: 'Now, some of the slaves seem to be revolting, and apparently with increasing frequency, are murdering the meddling medicos.' To prove his point, Szasz cites a report of a man who was suffering from mental illness and attacked and injured his mother. After this attack the man's parents initiated a commitment petition. Szasz's comment on this report is as follows: 'But the persons described in the above documents are not patients but criminals, most of whom cannot "return" to "productive" and "fulfilled" lives – if for no other reason than that they never had such lives.' We look in vain for Szasz to present evidence to support these assertions.

It is hard to comprehend such an attitude towards the lives of the patients referred to, and towards parents who have a mentally ill and violent son – from whom the law is reluctant to provide any relief until after he has assaulted or murdered. Szasz's only reply is that mental illness does not exist and therefore no-one is mentally ill. Morris has noted Szasz's tendency to see 'sharp lines where in fact there are fine gradations'.[14] He comments further on Szasz's 'cavalier treatment of a core issue, the difficult dilemma posed by our need to strike a balance between the risk of restraining responsible persons whose commitment is undesirable and the risk of not restraining persons whose commitment is desirable ... Now it may well be that much evil in this world has come about through interfering with people "for their own good", but Szasz seems content with leaving the matter there. It is a point that needs to be made, but at the beginning of discussion and not as the only discussion.'

Involuntary admission ultimately derives from social decisions not medical ones. In the United Kingdom the procedures are medical though the patients may appeal to a tribunal against the commitment decision. Despite the impressive list of problems and precautions surrounding such commitments, the legislatures and courts have continued to recognize the necessity of a procedure for confining those mentally ill persons who appear to be too dangerous to be left at liberty. These procedures are not foolproof; in retrospect, mistakes are made in both directions. But the case for accurate diagnosis and reasonably accurate prediction is much better than the critics claim. Most critics of diagnostic reliability cite older studies from the 1960s and early 1970s when less rigorous attention was paid to the construction of a nosological system which could elicit an acceptable measure of inter-rater diagnostic agreement.

Can psychiatrists make reliable diagnoses?

Present-day studies of diagnostic reliability indicate respectable figures of 80–90% agreement between raters for classifying illnesses into their major groupings such as organic brain syndrome, schizophrenia and affective disorder.[15] It is the intra-group ratings (which subtype of schizophrenia, or which specific neurosis or character disorder) that are less reliable. But these refinements are not essential for the task of commitment; assignment to the major category is the information which the court requires.

Critics often contrast the reliability ratings of psychiatric diagnoses with what they assume to be the better ratings of diagnoses in other branches of medicine. But there is in fact a base level of unreliability in all complex medical diagnoses. We find that pathology shades into normality − as in the recognition of cancer cells. And there is a base level of unreliability inherent in the technology (as where shadows on an X-ray film cannot always be resolved) and in laboratory tests which have a built-in margin of error. We are not suggesting that present psychiatric diagnostic reliability is fully satisfactory, or that there is no cause for concern − only that the concern has been exaggerated and misdirected.

For example, in a study of error and variation in the interpretation of electrocardiograms (ECGs) of fifty-three men aged 65–85, four cardiologists were asked to categorize the ECG patterns into 'normal', 'questionably abnormal' and 'abnormal', and also to offer specific diagnoses.[16] In addition, one observer was requested to assess the ECGs more than a year later. This observer upheld his own opinion on the second reading in 83% of his assessments. The level of agreement between the four observers was 84% for the three major groupings. However, this level of agreement dropped when specific diagnoses were offered, as follows: atrial fibrillation, 100% for three cases; myocardial infarction, 50% for ten cases; left ventricular hypertrophy, 49% for forty-one cases; myocardial ischaemia, 26% for nineteen cases. The author of this study cites a conclusion drawn by an earlier study that 'it is an illusion to believe there can be any arbitrary line between normal and abnormal tracings, or between abnormal and infarction tracings'. This level of reliability (84% for broad categories of normal and abnormal, 26–50% for specific diagnostic categories) is in the same range as psychiatric diagnoses.

In a study of levels of agreement regarding the presence or absence of chronic pyelonephritis (kidney damage secondary to chronic kidney infection) determined by intravenous pyelograms (in which a radio-opaque dye injected into the bloodstream is excreted by the kidney, thereby outlining the structure of the kidney on X-ray film), the intra-rater agreement between one radiologist's readings of the same X-ray films at two different times was 90%.[17] The inter-rater agreement between two radiologists was 80% when the 'undecided' films were left out of consideration. However, if the 'undecided' ratings were included as disagreements (since one radiologist offered decisions on ten pyelograms for which the other radiologist was 'undecided'), then the rate of agreement dropped to 68%. As indicated, these were the rates of agreement for assessment into global categories of presence or absence of disease. The rates of agreement for specific X-ray features, such as degree of dilatation, cortical thinning and loss of sharp calyceal cupping, dropped considerably to the levels cited above in the ECG study. The authors conclude: 'Thus, not pyelography alone but virtually every clinical diagnostic procedure must be examined critically to determine its variability.'

In a study of the influence of multiple readings on the problem of detecting and evaluating coal miners' pneumoconiosis, the X-ray findings of 55 730 miners were analysed.[18] The rate of agreement between local physicians and radiologists on presence or absence of pneumoconiosis was 75%. The films for which there was disagreement were sent to a second radiologist for an independent interpretation. The second radiologist agreed with the local physician in only 25% and with the first radiologist in 70% of these cases. The authors conclude: 'The extent of disagreement in the . . . readings for this group of miners' films in the first round of medical examinations is felt to be unacceptable. It is ironic that a system designed to determine proper compensation for respiratory disease is based on a test with a level of reliability lower than that which is acceptable for many other diagnostic techniques.'

In a report by the Royal College of Physicians and the Royal College of Pathologists on medical aspects of death certification, the findings are as follows:

Systematic inquiries into the accuracy of clinical diagnoses, which compare them with autopsy findings, consistently show that disagreement between the two is common: disagreement on the cause of death is found in 40–55 per cent of cases; disagreement on the main diagnosis and contributory conditions in 50–60 per cent. In a recent survey (with a high autopsy rate), clinicians and pathologists agreed that 15 per cent of cases showed diagnostic discrepancies that were considered to be 'clinically significant' (i.e. if the correct diagnoses had been suspected in life, different investigation and/or treatment would have been required).[19]

There is little need to labour the point by citing study after study. An ECG interpretation is so named because it is an interpretation, not a cold fact. This also applies to the reading of an X-ray film. It is a fact that there is a shadow or a blurring on the X-ray image, but the determination of what this represents entails a judgement. There is a degree of unreliability inherent in all such judgements. As Koran has written:

The reliability of many signs, procedures, and diagnostic and therapeutic judgements have never been studied. As for available studies, most are limited to small, unrepresentative samples of physicians, most fail to use statistics that correct for chance agreements, many do not disclose the participants' training and experience, and many examine tasks, such as interpreting electrocardiograms, performed in a manner different from that in which these tasks are performed in clinical practice. On the other hand, if the results of these studies are representative of the reliability of clinical data, methods, and judgements, there is little room for complacency.[20]

It is clear from examination of considerable evidence that psychiatric diagnoses, contrary to the assertions of the critics, are of the same order of reliability as diagnoses in other medical fields. This includes reliability in interpreting diagnostic procedures such as electrocardiograms, X-ray examinations and electroencephalograms which are ordinarily considered as providing greater reliability than other clinical judgements. Once again, attempts to demonstrate major differences between psychiatry and other fields of medicine ignore the consensus of evidence.

Although we have demonstrated the weaknesses of this attack on psychiatry, the valid question nevertheless remains: whether diagnosing as accurately as other physicians is good enough for the purpose at hand, namely, committing someone to hospital involuntarily. It is true that very serious decisions hinge upon diagnostic accuracy in all fields, such as in the case of physicians deciding whether coronary by-pass surgery is indicated in view of the severity of the coronary artery occlusions. But these are usually issues of mutual agreement between physician, patient and family and do not involve legal procedures which limit the freedom of a patient.

In fact, the information which the court needs relates much more to predictions of dangerousness than to details of diagnosis. This extended discussion of diagnostic reliability has been offered because the antipsychiatry writers have tried to impugn psychiatric credibility in general by attacking its diagnostic reliability. In addition, although the issue of the prediction of dangerousness is foremost, this prediction itself usually involves diagnostic considerations, and reasonably so, since the process of diagnosis takes into account present symptoms and behaviours, and evaluates them against family history, developmental data, school and work performance, and against other illnesses.

With regard to the specific question of whether diagnostic reliability as accurate as that in other medical fields is good enough for the particular purposes required by the court, we suggest that, in the absence of certainty, diagnostic reliability approaching 90% is sufficient to qualify as expert testimony and to allow the judge or jury to make a reasonable decision.

The prediction of violence

The second issue that must be addressed is the alleged inability of psychiatrists to predict violence. This too has been exaggerated. It has been based mainly on follow-up studies of the violence rate of patients released many years after they had been committed to state institutions.[21] The initial study was of patients released from maximum security hospitals under the Baxstrom decision.[22] Very few of these persons committed violent offences following their release. However, the rate of violence upon release of persons who had been institutionalized for many years following an initial determination of dangerousness is not relevant to the prediction of violence in the immediate and near future.

The conventional wisdom of thirty years ago was that mental patients were less violent than the general population.[23] This impression has apparently changed, and more recent studies have demonstrated that discharged mental patients have higher rates of arrest for violent crimes than the general population.[24] However the explanation for this reversal may well be that there is a small group of mental patients who had criminal records prior to their initial psychiatric hospitalization and who account for the increased rate of violence among discharged patients.[25] These findings can be interpreted as either supporting the argument for involuntary commitment (there exists a small group of mentally ill persons who have demonstrated that they are dangerous) or weakening the argument (persons are entering the mental health system who are criminals and belong in prisons). We accept that there is substance in both arguments.

There are a few studies that examine the immediate post-commitment behaviours of committed persons, alongside the behaviours of those who had a hearing and were not committed. Of course, these populations may not be comparable. What is required is a study which in a random manner sets free immediately half of those who were committed at a commitment hearing. But such a study is unlikely to be carried out. Yesavage et al.[26] did not find any significant differences in the incidence of assault between two groups of patients discharged after treatment from psychiatric hospitals, one group of which had been subject to committal proceedings. But Rofman et al.[27] in a study of Veterans Administration patients in Massachusetts, using rather different controls, reported a 0.41 probability that a patient under a compulsory order would commit an assault in the first 45 days of hospitalization compared with 0.08 probability in a control (non-committed) group. Hence whether commitment and confinement in hospital serve to decrease or to increase the risk of violence in patients suffering from psychiatric disorder is for the present open to a measure of conjecture. But given the degree of risk to which communities might be exposed and the probable ill-effects in the short and long term of failure to institute early treatment for acute mental disorders which could in the majority of cases be brought under control, one has to ask what proportion of communities would be prepared to give their assent to the legal prohibition of the involuntary admission and treatment of those who manifest the symptoms of acute psychotic illness.

Although accuracy of prediction of dangerousness remains unsatisfactory, the accumulated weight of the clinical and statistical studies of violence in mentally ill persons points to certain very clear indicators. These can be used by physicians in making their predictions so that the courts may make sound decisions. The best predictor of future violence is past violence, just as the best predictor of a future heart attack is one in the past. This is the single reliable factor that shows up time and again. However, a number of other factors are also correlated with violence; no one factor taken alone enables the physician accurately to predict violence, but the combination of several factors indicates a considerable risk.[28] These risk factors include age and sex (young men), evidence of mild brain damage, paranoid diagnosis, history of alcohol or drug abuse, and the existence of an identifiable target victim with whom the patient will come into contact. Other factors which probably ought to be taken into account include availability of weapons (particularly firearms, although any object can become a weapon) and the absence of a stable environment for the person to return to, if not committed. It becomes clear that the empirical establishment of risk figures still leaves the ultimate question unanswered. What is a high enough risk to justify commitment? This is a question for society to answer. It is psychiatry's task to improve the accuracy of information which it provides to courts of law.

It is essential to distinguish between assessment of risk factors and prediction. All management in medicine deals with statistical risk refined by consideration of individual features, especially in situations that are potentially perilous. The conceptual basis of this has not been clarified until recently. Some psychiatrists have not understood, any more than other physicians, that individual predictions are inaccurate. There is always a measure of uncertainty involved in individual conditions; statistical prediction for large numbers can be made fairly accurately. The issue is whether in events of low probability, the judge's prediction is better than the psychiatrist's. Statistically the most accurate course is to predict no violence. But this leaves the problem unsolved.

The other difficulty which vitiates prediction is that the likelihood of detection of violence, and the factors that serve to constrain violence, are unknown. How much is known about people who know they are liable to reincarceration for wrongdoing? How much violence committed by the subjects of the prediction studies has gone undetected?

As we have stressed, prediction of violence with a high degree of accuracy is not a simple matter and civil commitment is a very serious business. But so too is the risk to society of violence committed by a mentally ill person who has already provided good reason for others to believe that he might be dangerous. In the view of Szaszian libertarians the danger is illusory. Or insofar as it is real, any destructive or violent acts committed by those diagnosed as mentally ill should be punished since they are in no sense different from the antisocial acts of criminals. Mental illness and by implication mental suffering are non-existent: only bodies can be ill or diseased. To talk of mental disease is to commit a category mistake. Those designated as mentally ill are and should be held responsible. To admit them or treat them on an involuntary basis, whether or not their conduct is self-destructive or dangerous for others, is to violate their human rights. In other words the suffering and hardship inflicted on individual patients and society by disorders of the mind may all be readily eliminated by abolishing the concept of mental illness. This is a literally mindless theory regarding the nature of the phenomena with which psychiatrists deal. For it postulates the presence of structural or other lesions as the sole criterion of demarcation between disease and non-disease and so denies the status of disease even to that substantial proportion of indubitable physical illnesses in which no clear evidence for any kind of lesion has as yet come to light.[29] Such an elaborate myth disguised as a theory about the nature of mental disease can have no point of contact with the problems it purports impartially to investigate.

Insanity defence

A young man named Hwaetred became afflicted with an evil spirit. So terrible was Hwaetred's madness that he tore his own limbs and attacked others with his teeth. When men tried to restrain him, he snatched up a double-bladed axe and killed three men. After four years of madness and with emaciated body, he was taken by his parents to several sacred shrines. But he received no help. One day, when his parents were wishing more for his death than for his life, they heard of a hermit [Guthlac] on the isle of Crowland. They took their possessed son, with limbs bound, to the hermit.   (Felix: Life of St Guthlac)[29a]

Guthlac lived in rural England AD 674–714, in the period known as the Dark Ages. Yet this narrative offers, in its matter of fact way, some remarkable insights into social attitudes towards mental illness in a period often vilified as the depth of brutality, ignorance and superstition. First of all, Hwaetred's condition was recognized as mental illness. His deviance was not minor; it called attention to self. This is not a case of someone behaving a little peculiarly. He tore at his own limbs and attacked others with his teeth. When men, presumably neighbours and relatives, attempt to restrain him from hurting himself and others, he kills three men in his ferocity. Yet we do not hear of revenge or even an attribution of criminality or guilt. It would have been far simpler and safer to have hunted Hwaetred down and killed him at a distance as a wild beast, with spears or bow and arrow. Instead the neighbours try to restrain him, the usual procedure for violent madmen in primitive societies. After he kills these men, Hwaetred is left alone for four years, like Nebuchadnezzar in his madness. But when he is weakened by emaciation, his parents, not having abandoned hope despite all that has happened, have him bound and carry him to several healing shrines, but to no avail. The narrator gives us an insight into the anguish of parents of a madman: they were wishing more for his death than his life. But they hear of a hermit living out in the marshy wilderness who is renowned for his cures and are willing to make yet one more attempt for the sake of their son.

The understanding depicted here that madmen were not to be held responsible for their criminal activities, including homicide, finds expression in several of the medieval law codes. The Lombard Laws, written between AD 643 and 755, state that if a man goes mad and does damage to man or beast, the accustomed fine shall not be required from the family.[30] The Procheiros Nomos, published by the Emperor Basil I at Constantinople between AD 867 and 879, states that children under seven and madmen cannot be punished for murder.[31] Henry Bracton, writing a comprehensive legal treatise on English law in 1256, argued that madmen cannot be held responsible for criminal acts because they lack the reason to form intent.[32] In a recent article B. H. Westman has offered evidence that late medieval (fourteenth-century) English juries were aware of insanity as a motivation of crime and were permitted under law to pardon the mentally deranged.[33]

However, the obviousness of mental illness as providing exculpation for criminal behaviour is no longer accepted as it was in past societies. Questions regarding the insanity plea and criminal responsibility have recently become more controversial because of a general sense that the use of this defence has been abused. For example, the *Wall Street Journal* reported the case of a stockbroker who embezzled $16 million in funds from a small bank.[34] This man offered an insanity defence based on the claim that he was suffering from a mental illness called pathological gambling. As Morse points out the integrity of the criminal justice system is compromised by taking invalid claims seriously.[35]

The remedy most frequently mentioned for these abuses is to abolish the insanity defence altogether. In fact, the American Medical Association recently recommended its abolition in criminal trials. It justified this recommendation on the basis that the insanity defence invites continuing expansion and corresponding abuse and, as a result, 'inspires public cynicism and contributes to erosion of confidence in the law's rationality, fairness, and efficiency'. In its place, the AMA recommended statutes providing for acquittal when the necessary state of mind (*mens rea*) was lacking.[36] Yet it is important to sort out the abuses which a system permits from the general principles underlying that system. It is possible that if a system allows too much abuse, it is in need of drastic overhauling. But there is no system of government, of administration, or of voluntary association of human beings which is not subject to abuse. Presidents, prime ministers, senators, Members of Parliament, judges, lawyers, doctors, generals, policemen, labourers, barmen, husbands and wives all at times abuse the rules under which they have agreed to live and work. Kadish has argued, in support of improving rather than abolishing the insanity defence, that 'the insanity defence is scarcely the only feature of our criminal justice system which is badly administered in practice'.[37] He points out, for example, that in the United States 'inefficiency and inequity are endemic to a system committed to an adversary process but not committed to supplying the resources of legal contest to the typically penurious who make up the bulk of criminal defendants'. Kadish voices the hope that the lesson learned would not be to abandon the adversary method on that score, but to improve its operation.

In the United Kingdom the Butler Committee[37a] recommended radical revision of the insanity defence as advanced under the M'Naghten Rules. It also recommended abolition of the defence of diminished responsibility. But the proposals are unlikely to be enacted in the foreseeable future.

We are not complacent about abuses of the insanity defence, but think that they do not constitute sufficient grounds to abandon the principle itself – that is, that the concept of criminal behaviour requires *intent*, and that certain types of mental illness *may* interfere with a person's ability to form intent.

That criminal behaviour requires a mental state (*mens rea*) capable of intent, is a fundamental principle of Anglo-American law and is not at issue here, as this is how the law is at present written and interpreted. What is at issue is whether certain instances of mental illness are incompatible with the ability to form intent as this concept is used by the law. The *mens rea* requirement for culpability touches at the very foundation of the purposes of criminal law, which are generally considered to be deterrence, retribution (payment for fault) and rehabilitation. It would be unjust to punish someone who was not responsible for the occurrence of an unfortunate event, even a death. Imagine that a light switch is rigged up to a bomb such that when you enter a room and press the switch, ignorant of the sequence of events you are initiating, the bomb explodes somewhere else and kills a person. It would be unjust to hold you criminally responsible, although your actions were part of a chain of events leading to the death of a person. Further, imagine that you are seated in your car which is stationary at traffic lights. A large vehicle smashes into your car and propels it forward so that it runs over and kills a pedestrian. It would likewise be unjust to hold you criminally responsible for this death.

The question is whether the concepts of ignorance of the consequences of an action and of involuntary action, as exemplified in the two imaginary cases above, can be transferred to the actions of an insane person. Can we say, as though it is a matter of fact, that a mentally ill person is so cognitively impaired that he does not know what he is doing, or the consequences of his actions, or that he had no control over his actions? And is the question of whether a mentally ill person is *sufficiently* crazy, as Morse phrases it,[38] to qualify for special legal consideration, a medical or a social and moral judgement? In general, the question of 'How much is enough?' is usually regarded as one that must reflect social policy. However, the basis for this distinction must rest on some sort of psychological examination and understanding, if the *mens rea* concept of culpability is to have any meaning. With this in mind, we will build our discussion around two related questions. The first, as phrased by Feinberg,[39] is: When should we accept mental illness as an excuse? The second, as phrased by Morris,[40] is: What is the rationale for excusing the mentally ill?

Morris has pointed out the absence of a fully articulated and persuasive rationale for excusing the mentally ill. 'We are,' he writes, 'instead proferred language that captures our intuitions and little more: "it would be unfair to hold the insane responsible".'[41]

This is a critically important point, and some critics of psychiatry, such as Szasz, make the most of it. It is not self-evident to Szasz that the mentally ill should be excused their criminal actions. In fact, the contrary is self-evident to him, and he challenges others to provide a rationale for the insanity plea that goes beyond the 'it is intuitive' argument. But then Szasz proceeds to offer us other intuitively based values which we should accept with no better rationale. They include the proscription against murder and the apotheosis of liberty. Such values are integral to our Western culture as it has evolved over thousands of years, and we are therefore inclined to accept them as self-evident and of fundamental importance. But, we may well ask, whence comes the accepted rule that 'Thou shalt not kill' and whence come the inalienable rights to 'life, liberty, and the pursuit of happiness'? We can acknowledge that 'Thou shalt not kill' derives from the Ten Commandments, and is regarded by many people as being of divine origin. The same could not be said of 'life, liberty, and the pursuit of happiness'. But we might also require for ourselves a justification of 'Thou shalt not kill' more immediate than divine command.

When we look for more fundamental grounds for our codes of conduct and our highest values, we generally come up with two species of arguments: the intuitive and the pragmatic. Neither seems particularly compelling when subjected to logical scrutiny, and indeed, judging by many nations' and many individuals' behaviour, we could say that in many areas of the world there is no respect for liberty or the other person's life. The moral proscription against murder appears to be relative, not absolute. It is permitted, even encouraged, to kill the enemy in times of war and other forms of national conflict. It is permitted to kill in self-defence, and the state is permitted at various times to execute criminals. Yet despite these shortcomings of performance, we accept as intuitively obvious that, when feasible, 'Thou shalt not kill.'

If we search for social and pragmatic reasons for this rule, we encounter political philosophies which argue that the very foundations of human community as we value it would be destroyed if people went about killing each other freely, or whenever the risk of retribution seemed slight enough. It is held that peace and security are essential for the maintenance of society. Thus we find that in all societies there is a prohibition of killing fully invested members of that society. This prohibition does not always extend to slaves and other disenfranchised persons.

But is there a deeper rationale for not killing other than that it would make the conditions of living intolerable, or that we know intuitively that it is wrong? These are certainly not trivial reasons, but one searches in vain for a compelling justification, for a reason behind the reason. Finally, we have to accept that, as in geometry, certain rules are axiomatic. They are accepted as true and necessary.

If our justification for 'Thou shalt not kill' remains an intuitive or pragmatic one, what shall we say of liberty? It is clear that there are value systems, especially many with religious orientations, where liberty, far from being the highest good, is viewed as a positive evil. Liberty leads to licence and political anarchy, and to loss of the eternal soul. Western democracy tends to contrast liberty with tyranny and fascism, but democracy is not the only alternative to tyranny. There are others, such as an enlightened monarchy or a theocracy. There are also models on a smaller scale, such as tribal organization and monastic rule. The monastery is founded on the principle of obedience, not liberty.

Liberty is primarily a Western notion. We can trace its long and uncertain development throughout European history to the point we have reached today. Since we are the inheritors of this particular tradition, it is evident to us that liberty is the highest goal of political organization. Yet it is equally evident that liberty, like the prohibition against killing, is relative, not absolute. There are in fact many limitations to individual liberty, several of which are derived from the axiom that one's liberty must not intrude upon another's liberty. Thus, one is not free to pour pollutants and poisons into rivers and lakes, one is not free to build any type and shape of house anywhere one wants even if one owns the land, one is not free to travel about with smallpox, one is not free to shout 'Fire!' in a crowded theatre, and one is not free to advocate the overthrow of the government by force or the assassination of the head of state. Such limitations on individual liberty may be lamented but they are unavoidable if the greatest possible measure of freedom is to be vouchsafed to each and every member of society. The limitations serve further to illustrate the relativity of the concept of freedom. For although the evidence in defence of it is based in part on lessons extracted from the historical record, it is also strongly rooted in the intuitive judgment that liberty is a precious and fundamental human right and that its progressive curtailment beyond the minimal measures demanded to protect it would bring about fundamental changes in free societies and ultimately render them insupportable. Yet these arguments – compelling as they may be to us – might fail to convince someone reared in a different culture and whose ideas about society and the right to liberty start from different premises.

The insanity plea has a justification as strong as that of the prohibition against murder and considerably stronger than the argument for liberty. All these rest on the same sort of consideration. The justification of the insanity plea has a threefold basis. First it is intuitively obvious; second, it is a firm part of our tradition, dating back to Biblical times and extending to the present day, and it has been honoured in all societies investigated, whether primitive or 'civilized', which is not true of liberty; and third, since it rests upon certain basic assumptions of our concept of man, to remove the insanity plea is to undermine the foundation of our society.

It is difficult to provide convincing arguments for beliefs that are claimed to be intuitive. Yet here, as we indicated, there is an argument as sound as the argument against killing. The argument, essentially, consists of marshalling the evidence that all societies have acknowledged that the insane are not responsible for their criminal actions, just as they have acknowledged that intratribal killing cannot be tolerated. This acknowledgement can only be based upon the intuitive understanding that something is different about the insane which places them outside the law as it is understood to apply to criminal responsibility. Indeed, this understanding applies not only to the insane, but also to idiots and children. The designated age, the degree of idiocy, the extent of insanity may differ in the rules of different societies, but everywhere these three groups are held not responsible for their criminal actions. The rationale may be articulated or not; it would appear that the intuitive understanding precedes the elaboration of the justification, which is required only as a legal system develops a coherent philosophy.

Thus in our culture, criminal responsibility is elaborated in terms of intent and understanding. While these two concepts clearly do not apply to idiots and children, the critics of the insanity plea are quick to point out that a mentally ill person, for example a paranoid person, has both intent and understanding of the nature of his act, and therefore is responsible for it. They are correct in the letter of the argument, but not in the sense of it. For the justification according to intent and understanding is a *post hoc* argument employed to rationalize something which we know intuitively to be right. Lack of intent and lack of understanding do not adequately describe the condition of the mentally ill.

There is an additional condition which is universally recognized but evades description because it refers to the very vague but forceful notion of the self. We are *not* speaking of a reified substance, a thing, a ghost in the machine. We are speaking of a concept, as is liberty itself. We each have a sense of a self within us which is not based upon logic or any evidence other than what is self-evident. We have a sense of our self as having stability and continuity through time, and, by and large, extend this sense to other people too. We do not have to justify this sense of self, since it is immediately and intuitively obvious. Insanity is perceived as a disruption or change of this stable concept of selfhood; since the 'self' evades our attempts at complete description, so too does the alteration of this sense of self. But it is universally recognized. The fact that persons can simulate madness or that we have difficulty in knowing the boundaries of madness in no way invalidates our basic and intuitive recognition. Nor are we claiming that this 'intuition' is instinctive, although the presence of universal concepts does lend support to a structuralist argument. But we do not have to go so far. There are undoubtedly many bits of knowledge which we attribute to intuition which are derived from our shared cultural experiences. Either way the arguments for not killing, the value of liberty, and the insanity plea are all of a piece: they are either intuitive, or we show why society would break down without them.

Finally, can we say that society would break down without an insanity plea? Suppose society will *not* break down without it: we can also say that society will not break down without liberty. Thus the arguments proceed apace. The insanity plea is based upon the same concept of man having free will as is the value of liberty. Man is a willing, thinking, desiring and rational being. As such, and in order to maintain a social order, we choose to hold man responsible for his actions. The insanity plea *merely* acknowledges that there are some persons for whom this is not true, or does not apply. These are infants, idiots and the insane. The choice to delete this last category flies in the face of universal common sense and the tradition of civilized societies.

One concern appears to be that if mental illness is allowed to excuse criminal behaviour, the doors are opened to broader and broader applications of the insanity defence. This appears especially disquieting if psychodynamic considerations are permitted to exculpate criminal behaviours. Could we not claim that all of life's adversities – poverty, racial discrimination, abusive parents, unhappy marriages – play influential roles in determining human behaviour? The making of a psychiatric diagnosis, however, does not pre-empt all moral judgements. Psychiatry does not advocate the abandonment of historical judgement, but rather a modification of society's moral stance by elucidating the early origins of certain criminal behaviours – for example, the connection between suffering appalling violence in early life and adult crimes. This does not deny the general right and necessity for society to pass judgment and to deter, punish and rehabilitate. Practical as well as philosophical reasons lead us to hold some persons to be guilty. This is not a reason for withholding and rejecting the insanity plea in all cases. Kadish has summarized this issue in the following terms:

We may accept as a necessary evil – necessary, that is, given our commitment to a punishment system – the criminal conviction of persons whose ability to conform is somewhat impaired and still protest that it is unacceptable for a society to fail to make a distinction for those who are utterly and obviously beyond the reach of the law.[42]

Mental illnesses are only one class of conditions that may excuse one from criminal responsibility. The common feature of all such conditions is that the action was involuntary, therefore intent was absent, and consequently a *crime* did not occur – or else, if a crime, then a lesser crime (for example manslaughter rather than murder). The two major forms of involuntary action in mental illness are usually attributed to compulsion or ignorance. Yet much of the psychopathology of mental illnesses does not fit easily under the 'compulsion' or 'ignorance' categories, except by bending either the symptoms or the categories beyond recognition. Not every mental illness provides an excuse from criminal responsibility; the question is what the essential ingredients must be. Since the insanity excuse appears to be recognized in most societies, primitive and industrial, there must be some traits which are common to mental illness in all societies. These must be easy to recognize – easier to recognize than to write down, in the same way that it is simpler to point to a cow than to try to define or describe one. It may be that very many societies have no difficulty in recognizing the extreme cases and that it is only in our legally developed societies that the concept is pushed more and more in the direction of the non-psychotic deviant.

For no one claims that every action and every thought of a psychotic person is irrational. As Feinberg points out,

there are various crimes that can be committed by persons suffering from mental illnesses that can have no relevant bearing on their motivation. We may take exhibitionism to be an excuse for indecent exposure, or pedophilia for child molestation, but neither would be a plausible defense to the charge of income-tax evasion or price-fixing conspiracy. These examples show, I think, that the mere fact of mental illness, no more than the mere fact of physical illness, automatically excuses.[43]

It is difficult to specify what it is about certain aspects of mental illness that allow it to be an excuse for certain criminal actions. A legal code cannot anticipate the details of every conceivable insanity plea and even has trouble defining precisely the boundaries within which it will accept insanity as an excuse. This does not mean that it cannot recognize it when it sees it, or that it cannot develop a workable although incomplete description which encompasses the class of situations which are applicable.

The majority of mentally ill persons can proceed through daily activities such as sleeping, waking, dressing, eating, walking and watching television. Some do it as well as 'normals', others with varying degrees of incapacity, especially compared with their own performance before they became ill. Many persons with paranoid illness show very little, if any, intellectual or social deterioration over the years of their illness, and can function in goal-directed ways as well as everyone else. Yet, there is an area of their functioning and thinking which is clearly dominated by intensely held delusional beliefs which appear to colour their entire being.

In order for mental illness to serve as excuse, a close link must be seen between the condition of illness and the action. In the first place the linkage occurs when the condition, the illness itself, has taken over the personality of the person so that he does not appear to be the same person. It is easy to see in this context why other societies classify some forms of mental illness as possession states. In everyday life we assume that there is a sort of executive or autonomous aspect of the personality that both constitutes its core and gives it coherent direction. Whatever the philosophical difficulties, in ordinary life we think of being in charge of ourselves in a way which does not seem true of many mentally ill persons. It is partly this which we have in mind when we consider that certain forms of mental illness may excuse criminal behaviour.

The other condition linking mental illness to the insanity plea refers to the domain of resistible and irresistible impulses. In some manner, some forms of mental illness appear to entail either stronger impulses or weaker controls over these impulses. Thus, to tell a manic patient to go to sleep at bedtime, to stop talking incessantly or not to be angry makes no sense, since it must be abundantly clear to all who have contact with such a person that he *cannot* sleep, cease talking or moderate his anger. He does not behave this way because he is manic; this behaviour *is* the mania at a clinical level. We say that he *cannot*, recognizing not only that such a statement cannot be proved, but also that it involves a circularity. Our experience in observing and trying to treat manics teaches us that they *do* not sleep, stop talking or moderate their anger. And somewhere in the course of this experience we conclude that they cannot, just as we conclude that the paralysed person cannot move his paralysed limbs, although we may not have proof. Similarly the person with an agitated depression cannot stop worrying that he will never get better. How do we know? We base it on our experience, recognizing that we have introduced a leap of logic from 'does not' to 'cannot'.

To reach this conclusion is itself a difficult matter. The ascription of wilfulness and choice to such a person's action is hard to avoid. We base this upon our own subjective experience that we have choice over our own behaviour, that we act as we do because we choose to. Therefore we are prone to assume that the manic talks incessantly because he chooses to. Yet one need only spend a few hours, or a few days, with a manic to convince oneself that 'choice' appears to have little to do with the behaviour in question.

Freedom of will, mental illness and the rule of law

The issue raised at the end of the previous section demands further analysis, for the problems posed by the scope and limitation of the concept of mental illness are related to the unresolved contradictions and dilemmas inherent in the concept of free will as against determinism in human conduct. Some of the issues discussed more fully in Chapter 4 will be considered briefly from a new angle in this section.

When we use introspection to probe our inner mental life and experience we seem to discover choice and free will. But study of the behaviour of others yields convincing evidence for determinism. We have learned that their personalities have been shaped by their inherent genetic endowment and their familial and social circumstances during the formative years of childhood development. Moreover their behaviour is characterized by certain distinctive patterns so that within certain limits their conduct is predictable. If this were not the case, human relationships and the forms of social co-operation for which they are the essential preconditions would not be possible. Friendships are established, love affairs embarked upon, marriages contracted and individuals chosen for positions of higher or lower responsibility on the basis of forecasts from past to future behaviour. Such predictions may of course prove wrong, but if they were less often correct than in error, human co-operation and an orderly social life would have been rendered impossible.

That an individual can refute such predictions on being informed in advance of the behaviour he is expected to manifest does not constitute valid evidence against the element of truth in the determinist position. It is logically flawed in that it arbitrarily introduces a confounding variable irrelevant to the basic hypothesis under examination. Such prior information does not differ in essence from the disproof of the predicted result of an athletic contest by administering hypnosis or a drug to the participant with the best previous performance.

It is, however, the evidence (cf. Chapter 4) for the intimate and inextricable connection between mental states and brain processes, supported to some extent by specific relationships between certain anatomical regions and particular activities such as speech, memory and emotion, that constitutes the most powerful argument for the reductionist determinist position. It does not establish their identity but raises the possibility that in the light of further progress in neurobiology, the view that defends the independent existence of some mental processes will be progressively eroded.

This represents only one horn of the dilemma. The results of introspection constitute the other. Impressive as the gathering evidence that denies mental processes any independence or causal effect appears, it cannot be allowed wholly to override the subjective experience of the individual that he is free to make and vary choices and act on them and that he can expand the range of his freedom through better knowledge, control and direction of himself.

The riddle of mind–brain relationship remains unsolved. But the contrast between the mental life and conduct of the ordinary person and the individual who suffers from schizophrenia, manic-depressive disorder or a related form of psychosis – the disorders in which the insanity defence is most commonly involved – helps to liberate us from some of the seemingly irreconcilable contradictions posed by the problem of free will. For it shows those unaffected by illness to possess the freedom to choose and to act within wide limits; in contrast, those whose illness has distorted their perception of the real world and rendered their thought, language and actions irrational and beyond the reach of empathic understanding, can be perceived to have suffered a severe restriction of their freedom of will or to be bereft of it. Thus the person who suffers from schizophrenia is compelled to listen to and obey his auditory hallucinations and to adhere to delusional beliefs in defiance of all contradictory evidence adduced from the real world. He experiences his will as usurped by occult and hostile influences, his body manipulated, and his thoughts directed and intruded upon. Hence by defining as precisely as possible the realm of illness, psychiatry seeks to create an objective basis for the distinction between sickness and moral failure that separates the realm of ethics and moral judgment from that of mental illness. It is inevitable that there should be an area of overlap between them. It is of limited extent and in the characterization of the patterns of behaviour located in this territory, concepts derived from ethics and those drawn from psychopathology do not pre-empt or displace each other. Both are valid although they serve distinct purposes.

To set limits to the concept of mental illness that are as precise and valid as existing knowledge permits, is a desirable objective. For no society can be created without the assumption that its members are responsible for their actions and culpable for any infringements of its laws – those with certain forms of mental illness excepted.

Alan Stone made a similar point in more emphatic terms when he stated, 'the insanity defence is the exception that "proves" the rule of law – the insanity defence does more than test the law, it *demonstrates* that all other criminals had free will – the ability to choose between good and evil – but that they chose evil and therefore deserved to be punished'.[44] It would perhaps be more consistent with the argument pursued here to say that the forms of mental disorder in respect of which the insanity defence is justified help to 'validate' rather than 'prove' the rule of law.

Mental illness and the alleged encroachment on the realm of moral judgment

Waelder[45] has advanced the view that there is a 'common core' to the concept of mental illness centred on 'conditions in which the sense of reality is crudely impaired, and inaccessible to the corrective influence of experience – for example, when people are confused or disorientated or suffer from hallucinations or delusions. That is the case in organic psychoses, in schizophrenia, in manic depressive psychosis. Their characterization as diseases of the mind is not open to reasonable doubt.'

One can add that it proves difficult or impossible to empathize with such individuals, to understand their thought and conduct, and that the history of their past adjustment reveals a break in the continuity of their psychic life in the sense of Jaspers; the rift from reality and the irrational conduct manifest have arisen at a definable point in time and in most cases of psychotic illness thought and behaviour manifest features that are qualitatively distinct from those observable in an individual before illness. It is possible to comprehend a murder carried out by a jealous and possessive husband who discovers his wife in adulterous intercourse with another man – even though we find the husband's conduct repugnant. But a murderous attack by a schizophrenic on a woman who is a complete stranger to him, and whom he accuses of stealing his semen by occult means in order to give herself a child so that she can sue him for paternity payments, belongs to a world of reasoning, feeling and action that is beyond the reach of empathy.

The psychotic group of mental illnesses therefore provides the basis for a relatively clear line of demarcation between conditions in which the insanity defence can in general be validly advanced and other mental disorders in which it is clearly unjustified and inadmissible. The insanity defence has been abolished in some states in the USA but in most European countries a man who has killed during an undubitably psychotic illness will usually be judged 'not guilty' on grounds of insanity.

On the other hand most persons suffering from neurotic disorder will be held responsible for offences against the law in all countries. A man who commits a well-planned armed robbery will be unlikely to secure acquittal on account of a number of phobic or obsessional symptoms; no defence drawing upon psychiatric testimony would be justified. For the range of morbid impulses in those with neuroses is circumscribed and confined to the limited domains in which their symptoms are expressed. Compulsive urges to carry out violent acts are recognized by the person affected as morbid and virtually never put into effect. And contact with reality and insight are largely or wholly intact in neurotic subjects.

But it would be unrealistic to expect the line of demarcation to be unequivocally sharp. The young girl with anorexia nervosa who has repeatedly been in danger of bringing her life to an end through starvation and who shoplifts large quantities of food which she hoards until it putrefies, is in a quite different category from the other examples cited. It would be a justice feeble in compassion and imagination that failed to realize that such a person is helplessly driven by a morbid compulsion and is not responsible for the offences with which she is charged. At the least her illness ought to be regarded as a mitigating factor. A further contrast is provided by the man who has poisoned his wife to lay hands on the sum of money for which she was insured. A psychiatric diagnosis of personality disorder should not, and usually does not, pre-empt either a moral judgment or a verdict of 'guilty of murder' in such an individual.

It is inevitable that such a limited area of fuzziness should have become evident at the outer limits of those complex states of mind of uncertain origin in which psychiatrists have been prepared to advance an insanity defence. It is inevitable also that this development should have caused concern to many eminent lawyers. The distinguished English judge Lord Devlin[46] has complained that 'everywhere the concept of illness expands continually at the expense of the concept of moral responsibility'. Barbara Wootton has expressed herself in similar terms.[47] The shift from moralistic judgment to psychodynamic explanation was mockingly parodied by the young delinquent in West Side Story who sang 'I am depraved on account I'm deprived.'

One can take issue for a number of reasons with the criticism of the moral climate Lord Devlin sees developing in contemporary society. The change in mores he has detected is not in question. But it has in part made for greater humanity, tolerance and efficiency. We attribute general paralysis of the insane to syphilis and not to moral turpitude; the panic-stricken state of housebound housewives to a specific neurosis, 'agoraphobia', rather than cowardice; and the breakdown of pilots after 40 or 50 bombing missions to acute anxiety neurosis rather than weak moral fibre. The psychiatric diagnosis is not just more compassionate; it is closer to the truth. However, it cannot be denied that some undesirable consequences have resulted from the change in the moral climate of the developed countries. The insanity defence and kindred pleas have been rarely entered in recent years. At a time when prisons are everywhere bursting at the seams any influence exerted by the infrequent appearances of psychiatrists in courts of law can have played only an insignificant part. Controversial cases would have been even fewer but for the adversarial system which encourages defending lawyers and their expert witnesses to inflate the psychiatric and psychodynamic factors in the exculpation from responsibility of those who have committed serious crimes. The unexpected verdicts that resulted in a few isolated but notorious cases have exerted a disproportionate effect in discrediting the insanity defence and psychiatric testimony in general. A quite different situation obtains in Scandinavian countries, where psychiatric experts are not permitted to present evidence as adversaries acting for opposing sides of a case under trial.[48] The court instead receives a single psychiatric report from a commission of appointed experts. These reports are treated with great respect. They are authoritative and the findings are very rarely challenged.

Other factors are likely to have contributed to the changes to which Lord Devlin drew attention. The fading of religious belief and the failure of any secular system of moral teaching to gain a comparable authority has probably weakened the capacity for remorse about wrong-doing and the willingness to take responsibility for it. Psychoanalytic theory has exerted similar influences in the medico-legal sphere and on social attitudes. For its teaching has tended to obliterate the lines of distinction between normal, neurotic and psychotic states of mind. And as unconscious forces are believed to predominate in deciding behaviour in them all, and the seeds of neurosis and psychosis are held to be embedded in everyone, the concept of mental illness has been deprived of any clear meaning. The contributions of psychoanalysis have expanded the range of human tolerance and compassion and dispelled the illusion that individuals, whether criminal or models of virtuous conduct, can be regarded as governed by reason alone. But as it is also implicit that every person is liable in some circumstances to be overwhelmed by psychodynamic forces hidden from conscious awareness, psychoanalysis has helped to disseminate concepts that can be elaborated to absolve individuals from direct responsibility for unjustified aggressive and antisocial acts. In the wider social sphere credence has been given to the idea that a latent state of malaise derived from unresolved conflict is ubiquitous in the human unconscious, and this idea gains philosophical influence through its being ostensibly grounded in scientific observation.

Some of the indubitable achievements of contemporary biological psychiatry and neurobiology, and the future developments they portend, generate deterministic ideas regarding human behaviour from a different quarter. They have helped further to create a climate in which moral judgments are regarded as relative and subjective – metaphysical concepts such as intention and free will are discarded in favour of theories more readily tested with the traditional methods of science. It has become possible in recent decades to alleviate or cure an individual suffering from a psychotic-depressive illness with suicidal tendencies by a few weeks of treatment that includes an appropriate antidepressive compound. Similar results are commonly achieved in patients suffering from manic illness. And in a proportion of cases of neurotic disorder that have proved refractory over a period of years to treatments derived from psychoanalytic theory, the clinical picture and life situation of individual patients may be transformed by biological therapies. Such results must be largely achieved through effects upon the biochemistry of the cerebrum.

Moreover progress has been made in defining some of the structural and neurochemical correlates of learning and experience in experimental animals. And it can only be a matter of time before similar achievements are recorded in human neurobiology. Hope has therefore been ignited among some scientists working on this frontier that it will eventually prove possible to account for behaviour in normal and morbid mental states alike in terms of cerebral neurophysiology and neurochemistry. If so, the way should be open for defining brain mechanisms as the primary causes of all mental events and for providing a complete description of subjective mental experience and objective behaviour in the language of cerebral activity. Some imprecise psychological language that seeks to delineate human motivation, free will and emotion will have been rendered redundant.

This presupposes that advances in neurobiology and biological psychiatry are certain to succeed at some time in the future by formulating a wholly deterministic solution for the mind–body problem that denies to mental events any causal effects independent of some specific physical starting point. Now it is possible that specific chemical deficits or metabolic disturbances will prove to be the underlying causes of the major psychoses. Contributory factors of this nature may also be identified in relation to some forms of neurotic disorder. But there appears to be no scientific justification for extrapolating from such discoveries (which, probable as they may seem, have yet to be achieved) to simplistic reductionist solutions to the riddle of the relationship between brain and mind. That human autonomy, intention, free will and responsibility are realities rather than illusions, is validated not only by subjective experience but by observations of the course of human development which reveal their progressive unfolding. The phenomena of serious mental illness provide supportive evidence in that they serve to define with clarity what happens when the most specifically human faculties are impaired or undermined as in the case of the schizophrenic and manic-depressive psychoses. Understanding of rationality and affect, autonomy and the unity of integration of human personality can therefore be heightened by the study of such disordered states. Yet the contrasts between those suffering from a psychosis and those not so affected and between a schizophrenic or manic person during illness and after recovery are among the most powerful testimonies for the reality of mental illness.

On 15 November 1853, writing in the first issue of the *Asylum Journal*, later to become the *Journal of Mental Sciences*, Sir John Bucknill paid tribute to Pinel who had 'vindicated the rights of science against the usurpations of superstition and brutality; and rescued the victims of cerebro-mental disease from the exorcist and the goaler'. He goes on to refer to the fact that the physician was now to become the responsible guardian of those with mental disorders and must remain so 'unless by some calamitous reverse the progress of the world in civilization should be arrested and turned back in the direction of practical barbarism'.

His words may have been prophetic. The last 20 to 25 years have seen the closure or running down of a high proportion of the psychiatric hospitals in the countries of the Western world. The majority of the patients with long-lasting or chronic mental disorders have been discharged into communities unprepared or ill-disposed to receive them. The medical and social care they receive there and the accommodation with which they are provided is generally inadequate and isolated and many patients have ended up among the homeless and vagrant or as the anonymous and transient occupants of low-grade residential accommodation for the indigent. In all the countries in which these trends have been manifest a growing proportion of psychiatric patients have been imprisoned in recent years, often for trivial offences but in a minority for more serious ones. The USA, Great Britain and Italy provide the clearest examples of the deleterious effects exerted by these developments upon the health and dignity of those who suffer from mental illness.[49]

Penrose[50] pointed out that in European countries before World War II there was a high inverse correlation between the number of hospital beds and the number of prison beds. In other words, countries which made scant provision for the treatment of those with mental illness tended to have a disproportionate number of individuals incarcerated in prisons. During the past century countries which have advanced their standards have done so by adopting more compassionate and less punitive approaches to many forms of conduct previously considered as sinful and criminal.

We have argued in this section that the concept of mental illness has definable boundaries and that medical forms of care are appropriate and efficacious only in circumscribable portions of those who present a danger to society. But recent trends, if allowed to continue, can only culminate in a society in which prisons again contain a large proportion of those who suffer from mental illness because there is no appropriate alternative form of care or accommodation for them. If such a situation should materialize, the distinction between prison and hospital will become once again blurred or obliterated as it was 133 years ago when Bucknill held out optimistic hopes of a new era in which science and humanity would jointly seek to surmount the problems presented by morbid mental suffering. The hard-won and remarkable progress achieved by psychiatry, during the past half century in particular, will then have been set into reverse.

Notes

1. Mental illness, psychiatry and its critics

1. Szasz, T. S. (1974) *The Myth of Mental Illness*. New York: Harper and Row; Szasz, T. S. (1976) *Schizophrenia: The Sacred Symbol of Psychiatry*. New York: Basic Books; Szasz, T. S. (1971) *The Manufacture of Madness*. London: Routledge and Kegan Paul.

2. Lemert, E. M. (1951) *Social Pathology*. New York: McGraw-Hill; Goffman, E. (1961) *Asylums*. Garden City, New York: Anchor Books; Scheff, T. J. (1966) *Being Mentally Ill*. Chicago: Aldine; Rosenhan, D. L. (1973) On being sane in insane places. *Science*, **179**, 250–8.

3. Laing, R. D (1965) *The Divided Self*. Baltimore: Penguin; Laing, R. D. (1967) *The Politics of Experience*. New York: Pantheon Books; Laing, R. D. and Esterson, A. (1970) *Sanity, Madness and the Family*. Harmondsworth: Penguin Books.

4. Foucault, M. (1973) *Madness and Civilization*. New York: Vintage Books; Basaglia, F. (1980) Problems of law and psychiatry: the Italian experience. *International Journal of Law and Psychiatry*, **3**, 17–37; Basaglia, F. (1981) Breaking the circuit of control. In D. Ingleby (ed.) *Critical Psychiatry*, pp. 184–92. Harmondsworth: Penguin Books.

5. Lewy, F. H. (1914) Zur pathologischen Anatomie der paralysis agitans. *Deutsche Zeitschrift für Nervenheilkunde*, **1**, 50; Onuaguluchi, G. (1964) *Parkinsonism*. London: Butterworths.

6. Farrell, B. A. (1979) Mental illness: a conceptual analysis. *Psychological Medicine*, **9**, 21–35.

7 Roth, M. (1982) Dementia in relation to aging in the central nervous system. In: R. D. Terry, C. L. Bolis and G. Toffano (eds.) *Aging*, vol. 18, *Neural Aging and Its Implications in Human Neurological Pathology*, pp. 231–50. New York: Raven Press.

8. Stamler, J., Stamler, R. and Pullman, T. N. (eds.) (1967) *The Epidemiology of Hypertension*. New York: Grune and Stratton; Weiner, H. (1977) *Psychobiology and Human Disease*, Chap. 2. New York: Elsevier.

9. Roth, M. and Kay, D. W. K. (1955) Affective disorders in the senium. II. Physical disability as an aetiological factor. *Journal of Mental Science*, **102**, 141–50; Kay, D. W. K. and Roth, M. (1955) Physical accompaniments of mental disorder in old age. *Lancet*, **II**, 740–5; Hare, E. H. and Shaw, G. (1965) *Mental Health in a New Housing Estate*. Maudsley Monograph No. 12. London: Oxford University Press; Maguire, G. P. and Granville-Grossman, K. L. (1968) Physical illness in psychiatric patients. *British Journal of Psychiatry*, **115**, 1365–9; Hall, R. C. W., Popkin, M. K., Devaul, R. A., Faillace, L. A. and Stickney, S. K. (1978) Physical illness representing as psychiatric disease. *Archives of General Psychiatry*, **35**, 1315–20; Koranyi, E. K. (1979) Morbidity and rate of undiagnosed physical illness in a psychiatric-clinic population. *Archives of General Psychiatry*, **36**, 414–19; Hall, R. C. W., Gardner, E. R., Stickney, S. K., LeCann, A. F. and Popkin, M. K. (1980) Physical illness manifesting as psychiatric disease. *Archives*

of *General Psychiatry*, **37**, 989–95; Katon, W., Kleinman, A. and Rosen, G. (1982) Depression and somatization: A review. *American Journal of Medicine*, **72**, 127–35 and 241–7; Sims, A. C. P. and Prior, M. P. (1982) Arteriosclerosis related deaths in severe neurosis. *Comprehensive Psychiatry*, **23**, 181–5.

10. Fras, I., Litin, E. M. and Pearson, J. S. (1967) Comparison of psychiatric symptoms in carcinoma of the pancreas with those in some other abdominal neoplasms. *American Journal of Psychiatry*, **123**, 1553–62; Kerr, T. A., Schapira, K. and Roth, M. (1969) The relationship between premature death and affective disorders. *British Journal of Psychiatry*, **115**, 1277–82; Whitlock, F. A. (1976) Suicide, cancer, and depression. *British Journal of Psychiatry*, **132**, 269–74; Whitlock, F. A. and Siskind, M. (1979) Depression and cancer: a follow-up study. *Psychological Medicine*, **9**, 747–52; Lehrer, S. (1980) Life change and gastric cancer. *Psychosomatic Medicine*, **42**, 499–502; Brown, J. H. and Pareskevas, F. (1982) Cancer and depression: cancer presenting with depressive illness: an autoimmune disease? *British Journal of Psychiatry*, **141**, 227–32; Shekelle, R. B., Raynor, W. J., Ostfeld, A. M., Garron, D. C., Bieliauskas, L. A., Liu, S. C., Maliza, C. and Paul, O. (1982) Psychological depression and 17-year risk of death from cancer. *Psychosomatic Medicine*, **43**, 117–25.

11. Davison, K. and Bagley, C. R. (1967) Schizophrenia-like psychoses associated with organic disorders of the central nervous system: a review of the literature. In: R. N. Herrington (ed.) *Current Problems in Neuropsychiatry, British Journal of Psychiatry* Special Publication No. 4.

12. Scheff, T. J. (1966) *Being Mentally Ill.* Chicago: Aldine.

13. Gove, W. R. (1970) Socical reaction as an explanation of mental illness: an evaluation. *American Sociological Review*, **35**, 873–84. Also (1972), **37**, 488–90.

14. Praag, H. M. van (1978) The scientific foundation of antipsychiatry. *Acta Psychiatrica Scandinavica*, **58**, 113–41.

15. Nor is this a new phenomenon. Dwyer demonstrated this pattern in a carefully documented study of admissions to New York state hospitals in the last quarter of the nineteenth century. The admitting physician's notes provided copious details of the family's efforts to care for the mentally ill person at home. Dwyer, E. (1983) Psychiatric theory and practice in nineteenth-century New York. Paper read at 56th Annual Meeting, American Association for the History of Medicine, Minneapolis, Minnesota, 4–7 May.

16. Gove, W. R. (1970) *op. cit.*, p. 880.

17. Goffman, E. (1961) *Asylums*, p. 146. Garden City, New York: Anchor Books.

18. Wing, J. K. and Brown, B. W. (1970) *Institutionalism and Schizophrenia*. London: Cambridge University Press.

19. Rosenhan, D. L. (1973) On being sane in insane places. *Science*, **179**, 250–8.

20. Weiner, B. (1975) 'On being sane in insane places': a process (attributional) analysis and critique. *Journal of Abnormal Psychology*, **84**, 433–41; Spitzer, R. L. (1975) On pseudoscience in science, logic in remission, and psychiatric diagnoses: a critique of Rosenhan's 'On being sane in insane places'. *Journal of Abnormal Psychology*, **84**, 442–52; Crown, S. (1975) 'On being sane in insane places': a comment from England. *Journal of Abnormal Psychology*, **84**, 453–5; Millon, T. (1975) Reflections on Rosenhan's 'On being sane in insane places'. *Journal of Abnormal Psychology*, **84**, 456–61.

21. Bloch, S. (1978) Psychiatry as ideology in the USSR. *Journal of Medical Ethics*, **4**, 126–31; Bloch, S. (1980) The political misuse of Soviet psychiatry: Honolulu and beyond. *Australian and New Zealand Journal of Psychiatry*, **14**, 109–14; Scarnati, R. (1980) The

prostitution of forensic psychiatry in the Soviet Union. *Bulletin of the American Academy of Psychiatry and Law*, **8**, 111–13; Appelbaum, P. S. (1981) Law and Psychiatry, Soviet style. *Hospital and Community Psychiatry*, **32**, 601–2; Koryagin, A. (1981) Unwilling patients. *Lancet*, **I**, 821–4.

22. Rousseau, J. J. (1754) *Discourse of the Origin and Basis of Inequality Among Men*. In: *The Essential Rousseau*, trans. L. Bair, p. 151. New York: New American Library, 1974.

23. *Ibid.*

24. Rousseau, J. J. (1762) *The Social Contract*, trans. G. D. H. Cole, p. 5. London: J. M. Dent, 1913.

25. Illich, I. (1982) *Medical Nemesis*. New York: Pantheon Books.

26. Rousseau, J. J. (1762) *Emile, or On Education*, trans. A. Bloom, p. 85. New York: Basic Books, 1979.

27. Laing, R. D. (1967) *The Politics of Experience*, p. 10. New York: Pantheon Books.

28. Szasz. T. S. (1973) *Ideology and Insanity: Essays on the Psychiatric Dehumanization of Man*. London: Calder and Boyars.

29. *Ibid.*

30. Rousseau, J. J. (1762) *The Social Contract*, p. 53.

31. Russell, B. (1945) *A History of Western Philosophy*, p. 694. New York: Simon and Schuster.

32. Midelfort, H. C. E. (1980) Madness and civilization in early modern Europe: a reappraisal of Michel Foucault. In: B. C. Malament (ed.) *After the Reformation*, pp. 247–65. Philadelphia: University of Pennsylvania Press.

33. Maher, W. B. and Maher, B. (1982) The ship of fools: stultifera navis or ignis fatuus'. *American Psychologist*, **37**, 756–61.

34. *Ibid.*, p. 760.

35. Szasz, T. S. (1965) *Psychiatric Justice*, pp. 266–9. New York: Macmillan.

36. An English translation of Law 180 is found in the appendix to: Basaglia, F. (1980) Problems of law and psychiatry: the Italian experience. *International Journal of Law and Psychiatry*, **3**, 17–37.

37. *Ibid.*, p. 18.

38. Basaglia, F. (1981) Breaking the circuit of control. In D. Ingleby, (ed.) *Critical Psychiatry*, p. 186. Harmondsworth: Penguin Books.

39. *Ibid.*, p. 185.

40. Jones, K. and Poletti, A. (1985) Understanding the Italian experience. *British Journal of Psychiatry*, **146**, 341–7.

41. Papeschi, R. (1985) The denial of the institution: a critical review of Franco Basaglia's writings. *British Journal of Psychiatry*, **146**, 247–54.

42. Sarteschi, P., Cassano, G. B., Mauri, M. and Petracca, A. (1985) Medical and social consequences of the Italian Psychiatric Care Act of 1978. In M. Roth and R. Bluglass (eds.) *Psychiatry, Human Rights and the Law*, pp. 32–42. Cambridge: Cambridge University Press.

43. *Ibid.*, p. 345.

44. For a positive review of Basaglia and the Italian experience, see Mosher, L. R. (1983) Recent developments in the care, treatment, and rehabilitation of the chronically mentally ill in Italy. *Hospital and Community Psychiatry*, **34**, 947–50; Mosher, L. R. (1983) Radical deinstitutionalization: the Italian experience. *International Journal of Mental Health*, **11**, 129–36.

45. Hempel, C. G. (1965) *Aspects of Scientific Explanation*. New York: Free Press.

46. Praag, H. M. van (1982) The significance of biological factors in the diagnosis of depressions. II. Hormonal variations. *Comprehensive Psychiatry*, **23**, 216–26; Sachar, E. J., Asnis, G., Halbreich, U., Nathan, R. S. and Halpern, F. (1980) Recent studies in the neuroendocrinology of major depressive disorders. *Psychiatric Clinics of North America*, **3**, 313–26.

47. Rogers, M. P., Dubey, D. and Reich, P. (1979) The influence of the psyche and the brain on immunity and disease susceptibility: a critical review. *Psychosomatic Medicine*, **41**, 147–64; Pettingale, K. W., Greer, S. and Tee, D. E. (1977) Serum IgA and emotional expression in breast cancer patients. *Journal of Psychosomatic Research*, **21**, 395–9; Stein, M., Schiavi, R. C. and Camerino, M. (1976) Influence of brain and behaviour on the immune system. *Science*, **191**, 435–40.

48. Kaplan, R. D. and Mann, J. J. (1982) Altered platelet serotonin uptake kinetics in schizophrenia and depression. *Life Sciences*, **31**, 583.

2. Disorders of the mind and the role of medicine in historical perspective

1. Foucault, M. (1973) *Madness and Civilization*, pp. 269–71. New York: Vintage Books.

2. Scull, A. T. (1975) From madness to mental illness: medical men as moral entrepreneurs. *Archives Européennes de Sociologie*, **16**, 218–51; Scull, A. (1983) The domestication of madness. *Medical History*, **27**, 233–48.

3. Scull, A. T. (1975) *Op. cit.*, p. 221.

4. Jones, K. (1982) Scull's dilemma. *British Journal of Psychiatry*, **141**, 221–6.

5. Laing, R. D. (1967) *The Politics of Experience*, p. 11. New York: Pantheon Books.

6. *Ibid.*, p. 90.

7. Sontag, S. (1978) *Illness as Metaphor*, p. 35. New York: Farrar, Straus and Giroux.

8. The Bible (King James Version) (1977) Nashville, Tennessee: Thomas Nelson.

9. Temkin, O. (1973) *Galenism: Rise and Decline of a Medical Philosophy*. Ithaca: Cornell University Press; Jackson, S. W. (1978) Melancholia and the waning of the humoral theory. *Journal of the History of Medicine*, **33**, 367–76.

10. Kroll, J. L. (1973) A reappraisal of psychiatry in the Middle Ages. *Archives of General Psychiatry*, **29**, 276–83; Clarke, B. (1975) *Mental Illness in Earlier Britain*. Cardiff: University of Wales Press; Jackson, S. W. (1972) Unusual mental states in medieval Europe: medical syndromes of mental disorder: 400–1100 A. D. *Journal of the History of Medicine*, **27**, 262–97.

11. MacKinney, L. C. (1937) *Early Medieval Medicine*. Baltimore: Johns Hopkins University Press; Sigerist, H. E. (1958) The latin medical literature of the early Middle Ages. *Journal of the History of Medicine*, **13**, 127–46; Talbot, C. H. (1967) *Medicine in Medieval England*. London: Oldbourne.

12. *Isidore of Seville: The Medical Writings*, trans. W. D. Sharpe (1964) *Transactions of the American Philosophical Society*, New Series, **54**, part 2, 3–75.

13. Flemming, P. (1929) The medical aspects of the medieval monastery in England. *Proceedings of the Royal Society of Medicine: Section of the History of Medicine*, **22**, 771–82; Kealey, E. J. (1981) *Medieval Medicus*. Baltimore: Johns Hopkins University Press.

14. Amundsen, D. W. (1978) Medieval canon law on medical and surgical practice by the clergy. *Bulletin of the History of Medicine*, **52**, 22–44.

15. Kristeller, P. O. (1945) The school of Salerno. *Bulletin of the History of Medicine*, **17**, 138–94; Lawn, B. (1963) *The Salernitan Questions*. Oxford: Clarendon Press.

16. Kroll, J. L. and Bachrach, B. (1984) Sin and mental illness in the Middle Ages. *Psychological Medicine*, **14**, 507–14.

17. Bede: Prose life of Cuthbert. In: B. Colgrave (ed. and trans.) *Two Lives of St. Cuthbert*, p. 203. New York: Greenwood Press, 1969.

18. Bede: *A History of the English Church and People*, book II, chapt. 5. Harmondsworth, Middlesex: Penguin Books, 1974.

19. Neugebauer, R. (1978) Treatment of the mentally ill in medieval and early modern England: a reappraisal. *Journal of the History of the Behavioural Sciences*, **14**, 158–69; Neugebauer, R. (1979) Medieval and early modern theories of mental illness. *Archives of General Psychiatry*, **36**, 477–83.

20. As an aside, it is often overlooked that not only women but also men, as sorcerers, were prosecuted and executed. For example, at the Salem witch trials, one man was pressed to death and six were hanged (*Records of Salem Witchcraft* (1864), ed. W. E. Woodward, vol. 1 and 2. Roxbury, Massachusetts. Privately printed. Reprinted 1969). See also Graubard, M. (1984) *Witchcraft and the Nature of Man*. Lanham, Maryland: University Press of America.

21. Descartes (1641). Meditations on First Philosophy. In: R. M. Eaton (ed.), *Descartes: Selections*, p. 90. New York: Charles Schribner's Sons.

22. Hollingsworth, T. H. (1968) *Historical Demography*. London: Sources of History Ltd; Russell, J. C. (1948) *British Medieval Population*. Albuquerque: University of New Mexico Press; Herlihy, D. (1974) The generation in medieval history. *Viator*, **5**, 347–64.

3. The evidence from transcultural enquiries

1. Murphy, H. B. M. (1982) *Comparative Psychiatry*. Berlin: Springer-Verlag; Jablensky, A. and Sartorius, N. (1975) Culture and schizophrenia. *Psychological Medicine*, **5**, 113–24; Marsella, A. J. (1979) Cross-cultural studies of mental disorders. In: A. J. Marsella, R. G. Tharp and T. J. Ciborowski (eds.) *Perspectives in Cross-Cultural Psychology*. New York: Academic Press; Goldhammer, H. and Marshall, A. W. (1949) *Psychosis and Civilization*. Glencoe, Illinois: Free Press; Howells, J. G. (ed.) (1975) *World History of Psychiatry*. New York: Brunner/Mazel; Devereux, G. (1980) *Basic Problems in Ethnopsychiatry* Chicago: University of Chicago Press; Kroll, J. L. and Bachrach, B. (1982) Medieval visions and contemporary hallucinations. *Psychological Medicine*, **12**, 709–21; Westermayer, J. (1985). Psychiatric diagnosis across cultural boundaries. *American Journal of Psychiatry*, **142**, 798–805.

2. Murphy, J. M. (1976) Psychiatric labelling in cross-cultural perspective. *Science*, **191**, 1019–28.

3. Westermeyer, J. and Wintrob, R. (1979) 'Folk' explanations of mental illness in rural Laos. *American Journal of Psychiatry*, **136**, 901–5; Westermeyer, J. and Kroll, J. L. (1978) Violence and mental illness in a peasant society: characteristics of violent behaviours and 'folk' use of restraints. *British Journal of Psychiatry*, **133**, 529–41; Westermeyer, J. (1980) Psychosis in a peasant society: social outcomes. *American Journal of Psychiatry*, **137**, 1390–4.

4. Westermeyer, J. and Wintrob, R. (1979) 'Folk' criteria for the diagnosis of mental illness in rural Laos: on being insane in sane places. *American Journal of Psychiatry*, **136**, 755–61; Westermeyer, J. and Sines, L. (1979) Reliability of cross-cultural psychiatric diagnosis with an assessment of two rating contexts. *Journal of Psychiatric Research*, **15**, 199–213.

5. Murphy, J. M. (1976) *op. cit.*, p. 1022.

6. *Ibid.*
7. Westermeyer, J. (1979) Folk concepts of mental disorders among the Lao: continuities with similar concepts in other cultures and in psychiatry. *Culture, Medicine and Psychiatry*, **3**, 301–17.
8. Kroll, J. L. and Bachrach, B. (1982) Visions and psychopathology in the Middle Ages. *Journal of Nervous and Mental Disease*, **170**, 41–9.
9. Westermeyer, J. (1979) *op. cit.*
10. World Health Organization (1975) *Schizophrenia: A Multinational Study*. Public Health Papers No. 63. Geneva: WHO.
11. Rin, H. and Lin, T. Y. (1962) Mental illness among Formosan aborigines as compared with the Chinese in Taiwan. *Journal of Mental Science*, **108**, 134–46.
12. Murphy, H. B. M. and Raman, A. C. (1971) The chronicity of schizophrenia in indigenous tropical peoples: results of a twelve-year follow-up survey of Mauritius. *British Journal of Psychiatry*, **118**, 489–97.
13. Waxler, N. E. (1979) Is outcome for schizophrenia better in nonindustrial societies? *Journal of Nervous and Mental Disease*, **166**, 769–74.
14. Torrey, E. F., Torrey, B. B. and Burton-Bradley, B. G. (1974) The epidemiology of schizophrenia in Papua New Guinea. *American Journal of Psychiatry*, **131**, 567–73; Torrey, E. F. (1980) *Schizophrenia and Civilization*. New York: Jason Aronson.
15. Murphy, H. B. M., Wittkower, E. D., Fried, J. and Ellenberger, H. (1963) A cross-cultural survey of schizophrenic symptomatology. *International Journal of Social Psychiatry*, **9**, 237–49.
16. Varga, E. (1966) *Changes in the Symptomatology of Psychotic Patterns*. Budapest: Akademiai Kiado; Achte, K. A. (1966) The course of schizophrenic and schizophreniform psychoses. *Acta Psychiatrica et Neurologica Scandinavica*, Supplement 155.

4. A consideration of the mind–body problem and its bearing on the concept of disease

1. Scull, A. (ed.) (1981) *Madhouses, Mad-Doctors, and Madmen*. Philadelphia: University of Pennsylvania Press; Baruch, G. and Treacher, A. (1978) *Psychiatry Observed*. London: Routledge and Kegan Paul; Ingleby, D. (ed.) (1981) *Critical Psychiatry: The Politics of Mental Health*. Harmondsworth, Middlesex: Penguin Books.
2. Kleinman, A. (1982) Neurasthenia and depression: a study of somatization and culture in China. *Culture, Medicine and Psychiatry*, **6**, 117–90.
3. Moore, M. S. (1975) Some myths about 'mental illness'. *Archives of General Psychiatry*, **32**, 1483–97.
4. Szasz, T. S. (1976) Schizophrenia: the sacred symbol of psychiatry. *British Journal of Psychiatry*, **129**, 308–16.
5. Leifer, R. (1970) The medical model as ideology. *International Journal of Psychiatry*, **9**, 13–21; Leifer, R. (1964) The psychiatrist and tests of criminal responsibility. *American Psychologist*, **19**, 830–5.
6. Searle, J. (1984) *Minds, Brains and Science*, p. 17. Cambridge, Mass.: Harvard University Press.
7. Feigl, H. (1953) The mind–body problem in the development of logical empiricism. In: H. Feigl and M. Brodbeck (eds.) *Readings in the Philosophy of Science*. New York: Appleton-Century-Crofts; Ryle, G. (1949) *The Concept of Mind*. New York: Barnes and Noble.
8. Rorty, R. (1965) Mind–body identity, privacy, and categories. *Review of Metaphysics*, **19**, 24–54.

9. Greyson, B. and Stevenson, I. (1980) The phenomenology of near-death experiences. *American Journal of Psychiatry*, **137**, 1193–6; Irwin, H. J. (1981) The psychological function of out-of-body experiences. *Journal of Nervous and Mental Disease*, **169**, 244–8; Twemlow, S. W., Gabbard, G. O. and Jones, F. C. (1982) The out-of-body experience: a phenomenological typology based on questionnaire responses. *American Journal of Psychiatry*, **139**, 450–5; Greeley, A. M. (1975) *The Sociology of the Paranormal: A Reconnaissance*. Sage Research Papers in the Social Sciences (Studies in Religion and Ethnicity Series No. 90–023). London: Sage Publications.

10. Hobbes, T. (1651) *Leviathan*. In: E. A. Burtt (ed.) *The English Philosophers from Bacon to Mill*. New York: Random House, 1939.

11. Brandt, F. (1927) *Thomas Hobbes' Mechanical Conception of Nature*. Copenhagen: Levin and Munksgaard; Peters, R. (1956) *Hobbes*. Baltimore, Maryland: Penguin Books.

12. Hankoff, L. D. (1980) Body–mind concepts in the ancient Near East: a comparison of Egypt and Israel in the Second Millennium B. C. In: R. W. Reiber (ed.) *Body and Mind: Past, Present, and Future*. New York: Academic Press.

13. Van Peursen, C. A. (1966) *Body, Soul, Spirit: A Survey of the Body–Mind Problem*. London: Oxford University Press. See also Simon, B. (1978) *Mind and Madness in Ancient Greece*. Ithaca, NY: Cornell University Press.

14. Mora, G. (1978) Mind–body concepts in the Middle Ages. I. The classical background and its merging with the Judeo-Christian tradition in the early Middle Ages. *Journal of the History of the Behavioural Sciences*, **14**, 344–61; Mora G. (1980) Mind–body concepts in the Middle Ages. The Moslem influence, the great theological systems, and cultural attitudes toward the mentally ill in the late Middle Ages. *Journal of the History of the Behavioural Sciences*, **16**, 58–72.

15. Putnam, H. (1981) Mind and body. In: H. Putman *Reason, Truth and History*, p. 75. Cambridge: Cambridge University Press.

16. Burge, T. (1979) Individualism and the mental. In: *Midwest Studies in Philosophy*, vol. 4, *Studies in Metaphysics*. Minneapolis: University of Minnesota Press; Wilson, M. D. (1980) Body and mind from a Cartesian point of view. In: R. W. Reiber (ed.) *Body and Mind*. New York. Academic Press.

17. Popper, K. R. and Eccles, J. C. (1977) *The Self and Its Brain*. Berlin: Springer-Verlag.

18. Eccles, J. C. (1976) Brain and free will. In: G. G. Globus, G. Maxwell and I. Savodnik. (eds.) *Consciousness and the Brain*. New York, Plenum Press. See also Savage, C. W. (1976) An old ghost in a new body. *Op. cit.*; Wilson, J. A. (1981) Eccles's physiological evidence for a self-conscious mind. *Brain, Behaviour and Evolution*, **18**, 33–40.

19. Schopenhauer, A. (1813) *On the Fourfold Root of the Principle of Sufficient Reason*, trans. Mme Karl Hillebrand (from the 3rd edn, 1864), p. 169. London: George Bell and Sons, 1981.

20. Snyder, S. (1982) Neurotransmitters and CNS disease: schizophrenia. *Lancet*, **II**, 970–4.

21. Watkins, L. R. and Mayer, D. J. (1982) Organization of endogenous opiate and nonopiate pain control systems. *Science*, **216**, 1185–92; Kosterlitz, H. W. (1979) Endogenous opioid peptides and the control of pain. *Psychological Medicine*, **9**, 1–4.

22. Sperry, R. W. (1977) Forebrain commissurotomy and conscious awareness. *Journal of Medicine and Philosophy*, **2**, 101–26; Gazzaniga, M. S. (1970) *The Bisected Brain*. New York: Appleton-Century-Crofts; Sperry, R. W. (1961) Cerebral organization and behaviour. *Science*, **133**, 1749–57; Marx, J. L. (1983) The two sides of the brain. *Science*, **220**, 488–90.

23. Praag, H. M. van (1982) The significance of biological factors in the diagnosis of

depressions. I. Biochemical variables. *Comprehensive Psychiatry*, **23**, 124–35; Gur,R. E., Gur, R. C., Skolnick, B. E. *et al.* (1985) Brain function in psychiatric disorders. *Archives of General Psychiatry*, **42**, 329–34.

24. Heston, L. L. (1966) Psychiatric disorders in foster home reared children of schizophrenic mothers. *British Journal of Psychiatry*, **112**, 819–25; Gottesman, I. I. and Shields, J. (1982) *Schizophrenia: The Epigenetic Puzzle*. Cambridge: Cambridge University Press; Bohman, M., Cloninger, C. R., von Knorring, A. L. *et al.* (1979) An adoption study of somatiform disorders. II. Cross-fostering analysis and genetic relationship to alcoholism and criminality. *Archives of General Psychiatry*, **41**, 872–8.

25. Smart, J. J. C. (1971) Sensations and brain processes. In: D. M. Rosenthal (ed.) *Materialism and the Mind–Body Problem*, p. 55. Englewood Cliffs, NJ: Prentice-Hall.

26. Polten, E. P. (1973) *Critique of the Psycho-Physical Identity Theory*, p. xii. The Hague: Mouton.

27. Smith, G. P. and Gibbs, J. (1976) Cholecystokinin and satiety: theoretic and therapeutic implications. In: D. Novin, W. Wynwicka and G. Bray (ed.) *Hunger: Brain Mechanisms and Clinical Implications*. New York: Raven Press.

28. Traskman-Bendz, L., Asberg, M. and Bertilsson, L. (1981) Serotonin and noradrenaline uptake inhibitors in the treatment of depression: relationship to 5-HIAA in spinal fluid. *Acta Psychiatrica Scandinavica*, Supplement 290, **63**, 209–18; Brown, G. L., Ebert, M. H., Goyer, P. F., Jimerson, D. C., Klein, W. J., Bunney, W. E. and Goodwin, F. K. (1982) Aggression, suicide, and serotonin: relationships to CSF amine metabolites. *American Journal of Psychiatry*, **139**, 741–6; Ostroff, R. Giller, E., Bonese, K., Ebersole, E., Harkness, L. and Mason, J. (1982) Neuroendocrine risk factors of suicidal behaviour. *American Journal of Psychiatry*, **139**, 1323–5; Traskman, L., Asberg, M., Bertilsson, L. *et al.* (1981) Monoamine metabolites in cerebrospinal fluid and suicidal behaviour. *Archives of General Psychiatry*, **38**, 631–6.

29. Wulff, H. R. (1981) *Rational Diagnosis and Treatment*. Oxford. Blackwell Scientific.

30. Sackett, D. L. (1977) Book review of Edmond A. Murphy: *The Logic of Medicine. Journal of Medicine and Philosophy*, **2**, 71–6.

5. Medical and alternative models of disease

1. Sokal, R. (1974) Classification: purposes, principles, progress, prospects. *Science*, **185**, 1115–23; Kendell, R. E. (1975) *The Role of Diagnosis in Psychiatry*. Oxford: Blackwell Scientific.

2. The passage is translated in MacKinney, L. C. (1934) Tenth-century medicine as seen in the Historia of Richer of Rheims. *Bulletin of the Institute of the History of Medicine*, **2**, 347–75.

3. *Ibid.*

4. McHugh, P. R. and Slavney, P. R. (1982) Methods of reasoning in psychopathology: conflict and resolution. *Comprehensive Psychiatry*, **23**, 197–215. See also McHugh, P. R. and Slavney, P. R. (1983) *The Perspectives of Psychiatry*. Baltimore: Johns Hopkins University Press.

5. Temkin, O. (1973) *Galenism: Rise and Decline of a Medical Philosophy*. Ithaca: Cornell University Press; McVaugh, M. (1969) Quantified medical theory and practice at four-theenth century Montpellier. *Bulletin of the History of Medicine*, **43**, 397–410.

6. Graubard, M. (1964) *Circulation and Respiration: The Evolution of an Idea*, p. 176. New York: Harcourt, Brace and World.

7. Hoffman, F. (1695) *Fundamenta Medicinae*, trans. L. S. King. London: Macdonald, 1975.

8. Brown, T. M. (1974) From mechanism to vitalism in eighteenth-century English

physiology. *Journal of the History of Biology*, **7**, 179–216.

9. Weiner, H. (1978) The illusion of simplicity: the medical model revisited. *American Journal of Psychiatry*, **135** (Supplement), 27–33. See also Penn, M. and Dworkin, M. (1976) Robert Koch and two visions of microbiology. *Bacteriological Reviews*, **40**, 276–83.

10. Eisenberg, L. (1977) Psychiatry and society: a sociobiologic synthesis. *New England Journal of Medicine*, **296**, 903–10.

11. Carroll, B. J., Feinberg, M., Greden, J. F. *et al.* (1981) A specific laboratory test for the diagnosis of melancholia. *Archives of General Psychiatry*, **38**, 15–22.

12. Rogers, M. P., Dubey, D. and Reich, P. (1979) The influence of the psyche and the brain on immunity and disease susceptibility: a critical review. *Psychosomatic Medicine*, **41**, 147–64; Locke, S. E., Kraus, L., Leserman, J. *et al.* (1984) Life change stress, psychiatric symptoms, and natural killer cell activity. *Psychosomatic Medicine*, **46**, 441–53.

13. Powell, G. F., Brasil, J. A. and Blizzard, R. M. (1967) Emotional deprivation and growth retardation simulating idiopathic hypopituitarism. *New England Journal of Medicine*, **276**, 1271–8 and 1279–83; Krieger, I. and Mellinger, D. C. (1971) Pituitary function in the deprivation syndrome. *Journal of Pediatrics*, **79**, 216; Money, J. and Annecillo, C. (1976) IQ changes following change of domicile in the syndrome of reversible hyposomatotropinism (psychosocial dwarfism). *Psychoneuroendocrinology*, **1**, 427–9; Money, J. and Werlwas, J. (1976) *Folie à deux* in the parents of psychosocial dwarfs: two cases. *Bulletin of the Academy of Psychiatry and the Law*, **4**, 351–62; Money, J. (1977) The syndrome of abuse dwarfism. *American Journal of Diseases of Children*, **131**, 508–13.

14. Weiner, H. (1978) The illusion of simplicity: the medical model revisited. *American Journal of Psychiatry*, **135** (Supplement), 27–33.

15. Engel, G. E. (1977) The need for a new medical model: a challenge for biomedicine. *Science*, **196**, 129–36.

16. *Ibid.*

17. Engel, G. L. (1980) The clinical application of the biopsychosocial model. *American Journal of Psychiatry*, **137**, 535–44.

18. Gottesman, I. I. and Shields, J. (1982) *Schizophrenia: The Epigenetic Puzzle*. Cambridge: Cambridge University Press; Kendler, K. S., Masterson, C. C., Ungaro, R. and Davis, K. L. (1984) A family history study of schizophrenia-related personality disorders. *American Journal of Psychiatry*, **141**, 424–7.

19. For a critique of this position, see: Pies, R. (1979) On myths and countermyths: more on Szaszian fallacies. *Archives of General Psychiatry*, **35**, 139–44.

20. Jerison, H. J. (1973) *Evolution of the Brain and Intelligence*. New York: Academic Press; Jerison, H. J. (1977) Evolution of the brain. In: M. C. Wittrock (ed.) *The Human Brain*, p. 54. Englewood Cliffs, NJ: Prentice-Hall. See also Alexander, R. D. (1979). *Darwinism and Human Affairs*. Seattle: University of Washington Press.

21. Snyder, S. H. (1982) Neurotransmitters and CNS disease: schizophrenia. *Lancet*, **II**, 970–4; Stevens, J. R. (1982) The neuropathology of schizophrenia. *Psychological Medicine*, **12**, 695–700.

22. Praag, H. M. van (1982) The significance of biological factors in the diagnosis of depressions. I. Biochemical variables. *Comprehensive Psychiatry*, **23**, 124–35; II. Hormonal variations. *Comprehensive Psychiatry*, **24**, 216–26.

23. Fabrega, H. Jr (1975) The position of psychiatry in the understanding of human disease. *Archives of General Psychiatry*, **32**, 1500–12.

24. Toulmin, S. (1977) The multiple aspects of mental health and mental disorders. *Journal of Medicine and Philosophy*, **2**, 191–6.
25. Bebbington, P. E., Hurry, J. and Tennant, C. (1980) Recent advances in the epidemiological study of minor psychiatric disorders. *Journal of the Royal Society of Medicine*, **73**, 315–18; Tennant, C., Bebbington, P. E. and Hurry, J. (1981) The natural history of neurotic illness in the community: demographic and clinical predictors of remission. *Australian and New Zealand Journal of Psychiatry*, **15**, 111–16; Bebbington, P. E., Tennant, C. and Hurry, J. (1981) Adversity and the nature of psychiatric disorder in the community. *Journal of Affective Disorders*, **3**, 345–66.
26. Mechanic, D. (1977) Illness behaviour, social adaptation, and the management of illness. *Journal of Nervous and Mental Disease*, **165**, 79–87.
27. David, G. B. (1957) The pathological anatomy of the schizophrenias. In: D. Richter (ed.) *Schizophrenia: Somatic Aspects*, pp. 93–130. Oxford: Pergamon Press; Shakow, D. (1946) *Nature of Deterioration in Schizophrenic Conditions*. Nervous and Mental Disease Monographs No. 70. New York: Coolidge Foundation.
28. Rousseau, G. S. (1980) Psychology. In G. S. Rousseau and R. Porter (eds.) *The Ferment of Knowledge: Studies in the Historiography of Eighteenth-Century Science*, p. 163. Cambridge: Cambridge University Press.
29. Sarbin, T. R. (1967) On the futility of the proposition that some people should be labelled 'mentally ill'. *Journal of Consulting Psychology*, **31**, 447–53; Scheff, T. J. (1966) *Being Mentally Ill*. Chicago: Aldine; Sarbin, T. R. and Juhasz, J. B. (1982) The concept of mental illness: an historical perspective. In: I. Al-Issa (ed.) *Culture and Psychopathology*. Baltimore: University Park Press.
30. Peele, S. (1981) Reductionism in the psychology of the eighties. *American Psychologist*, **36**, 807–18. See also Searle, J. (1984) *Minds, Brains and Science* (Cambridge, Mass., Harvard University Press) for a discussion of this point.
31. Blumer, D. and Migeon, C. (1975) Hormones and hormonal agents in the treatment of aggression. *Journal of Nervous and Mental Disease*, **160**, 127–37; Lloyd, C. W. and Weisz, J. (1975) Hormones and aggression. In: W. S. Fields and W. H. Sweet (eds.) *Neural Bases of Violence and Aggression*. St Louis: Warren H. Green; Hitchcock, E. (1979) Amygdalotomy for aggression. In: M. Sandler (ed.) *Psychopharmacology of Aggression*. New York: Raven Press; Sheard, M. H. (1979) Testosterone and aggression. In: M. Sandler (ed.) *op. cit.*; Sandler, M. (ed.) (1979) *Psychopharmacology of Aggression*. New York: Raven Press; Monroe, R. R. (1970) *Episodic Dyscontrol Disorders*. Cambridge, Mass.: Harvard University Press.
32. Geschwind, N. (1975) The clinical setting of aggression in temporal lobe epilepsy. In: W. S. Fields and W. H. Sweet (eds.) *Neural Bases of Violence and Aggression*. St Louis: Warren H. Green; Fields, W. S. and Sweet, W. H. (eds.) (1975) *Neural Bases of Violence and Aggression*: St Louis: Warren H. Green; Bear, D. M. and Fedio, P. (1977) Quantitative analysis of interictal behaviour in temporal lobe epilepsy. *Archives of Neurology*, **34**, 454–67; Blumer, D. and Benson, D. F. (1982) Psychiatric manifestations of epilepsy. In: D. F. Benson and D. Blumer (eds.) *Psychiatric Aspects of Neurologic Disease*, vol. 2. New York: Grune and Stratton; Herrington, R. N. (1969) The personality in temporal lobe epilepsy. *British Journal of Psychiatry*, Special Publication No. 4, pp. 70–6; Mungas, D. (1982) Interictal behaviour abnormality in temporal lobe epilepsy. *Archives of General Psychiatry*, **39**, 108–11; Lewis, D, O., Pincus, J. H., Shanok, S. S. and Glaser, G. H. (1982) Psychomotor epilepsy and violence in a group of incarcerated adolescent boys. *American Journal of Psychiatry*, **139**, 882–7.

33. Margoles, J. (1980) The concept of mental illness: a philosophical examination. In: B. A. Brody and H. T. Engelhardt, Jr (eds.) *Mental Illness: Law and Public Policy*, p. 3. Amsterdam: D. Reidel.

34. Cadoret, R. J. (1982) Genotype–environment interaction in antisocial behavior. *Psychological Medicine*, **12**, 235–9; Schulsinger, F. (1972) Psychopathy: heredity and environment. *International Journal of Mental Health*, **1**, 190–206; Crowe, R. R. (1974) An adoption study of antisocial personality. *Archives of General Psychiatry*, **31**, 785–91; Cattell, R. B. (1982) *The Inheritance of Personality and Ability*. New York: Academic Press; Hutchings, B. and Mednick, S. A. (1977) Criminality in adoptees and their adoptive and biological parents: a pilot study. In S. A. Mednick and K. O. Christanson (eds.) *Biosocial Bases of Criminal Behavior*, pp. 127–41. New York: Garden Press; Mednick, S. A., Gabrielli, W. F. and Hutchings, B. (1984) Genetic influences in criminal convictions: evidence from an adoption cohort. *Science*, **224**, 891–4. See also the controversy regarding this last article in letters to the editor by L. J. Kamin (p. 983) and L. E. Moses (pp. 983–4) and a reply by Mednick, Gabrielli and Hutchings. *Science* (1984), **227**, 983–9.

35. Bruner, J. S. (1968) The Freudian concept of man and the continuity of nature. In: M. Brodbeck (ed.) *Readings in the Philosophy of the Social Sciences*, p. 709. New York: Macmillan.

36. Klerman, G. L. (1977) Mental illness, the medical model, and psychiatry. *Journal of Medicine and Philosophy*, **2**, 220–43.

6. Social, ethical and philosophical aspects of involuntary hospitalization and the insanity defence

1. Hilary Putnam (*Reason, Truth and History*. Cambridge University Press, 1981, p. 128) correctly points out that 'the distinction [between fact and value] is at the very least hopelessly fuzzy because factual statements themselves, and the practices of scientific inquiry upon which we rely to decide what is and what is not a fact, presupposes values'. Our own discussion of cultural influences on concepts of illness bears this in mind. Nevertheless, there is a sense in common usage by which one can make a distinction between beliefs for which we have evidence which is reproducible and beliefs which are based on our feelings and attitudes. It is in this common-sense meaning that we draw a distinction between facts and values.

2. State laws governing civil commitment (1979) *Mental Disability Law Reporter*, **3**, 206–14.

3. Pope, H. G. Jr, Jonas, J. M. and Jones, B. (1982) Factitious psychosis: phenomenology, family history, and long-term outcome of nine patients. *American Journal of Psychiatry*, **139**, 1480–3.

4. Cutler, N. R. and Post, R. M. (1982) Life course of illness in untreated manic-depressive patients. *Comprehensive Psychiatry*, **23**, 101–15; Tsuang, M. T. and Woolson, R. F. (1977) Mortality in patients with schizophrenia, mania, and depression, and surgical conditions. *British Journal of Psychiatry*, **130**, 162–6; Black, D. W., Warrack, G. and Winokur, G. (1985) Excess mortality among psychiatric patients. *Journal of the American Medical Association*, **253**, 58–61.

5. Stone, A. A. (1982) Psychiatric abuse and legal reform: two ways to make a bad situation worse. *International Journal of Law and Psychiatry*, **5**, 9–28.

6. Hewetson, J. (1975) Homeless people as an at-risk group. *Proceedings of the Royal Society of Medicine*, **68**, 9–13; Asander, H. (1980) A field investigation of homeless men in

Stockholm. *Acta Psychiatrica Scandinavica*, Supplement 281; Baxter, E. and Hopper, K. (1981) *Private Lives/Public Spaces*. New York: Community Services Society; Bassuk, E. L., Rubin, L. and Lauriat, A. (1984) Is homelessness a mental health problem? *American Journal of Psychiatry*, **141**, 1546–50; Kroll, J. L., Carey, K., Hagedorn, D., Fire Dog, P. and Benevides, E. (1986) A survey of homeless adults in urban emergency shelters. *Hospital and Community Psychiatry*, in press.

7. Kroll, J. L. and Kisch, J. (1978) The managerial revolution in psychiatry. *Man and Medicine*, **3**, 153–200.

8. As a sad postscript, we learned, just prior to this book going to press, that this young woman committed suicide with a drug overdose.

9. Sainsbury, P. (1956) *Suicide in London*. New York: Basic books; Seager, C. P. and Flood, R. A. (1965) Suicide in Bristol. *British Journal of Psychiatry*, **111**, 919–32; Tuckman, J. and Youngman, W. F. (1968) A scale for assessing suicide risk of attempted suicides. *Journal of Clinical Psychology*, **24**, 17–19; Buglass, D. and Horton, J. (1974) A scale for predicting subsequent suicidal behaviour. *British Journal of Psychiatry*, **124**, 573–8; Beck, A. T., Resnik, H. L. P. and Lettieri, D. J. (eds.) (1974) *The Predictions of Suicide*. Bowie, Maryland: Charles Press; Kovacs, M., Beck, A. T. and Weissman, A. (1975) Hopelessness: an indication of suicide risk. *Suicide*, **5**, 98–103; Bagley, C., Jacobson, S. and Rehin, A. (1976) Completed suicide: a taxonomic analysis of clinical and social data. *Psychological Medicine*, **6**, 429–38; Pierce, D. W. (1981) The predictive validation of a suicide intent scale: a five year follow-up. *British Journal of Psychiatry*, **139**, 391–6; Borg, S. E. and Stahl, M. (1982) Prediction of suicide: a prospective study of suicides and controls among psychiatric patients. *Acta Psychiatrica Scandinavica*, **65**, 221–32; Ostroff, R., Giller, E., Bonese, K., Ebersole, E., Harkness, L. and Mason, J.(1982) Neuroendocrine risk factors of suicidal behaviour. *American Journal of Psychiatry*, **139**, 1323–5; Kaplan, R. D., Kottler, D. B. and Frances, A. J. (1982) Reliability and rationality in the prediction of suicide. *Hospital and Community Psychiatry*, **33**, 212–15; Roy, A. (1982) Risk factors for suicide in psychiatric patients. *Archives of General Psychiatry*, **39**, 1089–95; Pokorny, A. D. (1983) Prediction of suicide in psychiatric patients. *Archives of General Psychiatry*, **40**, 249–57; Mackenzie, T. B. and Popkin, M. K. (1985) Suicide in the medical patient. In: D. Schubert (ed.) *Depression in the Medically Ill*. New York: Plenum Press (in press).

10. *Statistical Abstract of the United States: 1978*, 99th ed. Washington DC: US Bureau of the Census; *Mortality Statistics Review of the Registrar General on Death by Cause, Sex and Age in England and Wales, 1980* (1982) Series DH2, No. 7 Crown Copyright.

11. Steadman, H. J. (1980) The right not to be a false positive: problems in the application of the dangerousness standard. *Psychiatric Quarterly*, **52**, 84–99.

12. Ennis, B. J. and Litwack, T. R. (1974) Psychiatry and the presumption of expertise: flipping coins in the courtroom. *California Law Review*, **62**, 693–752.

13. Szasz, T. (1982) Bang bang, you're sick: shooting the shrink. *The New Republic* 16 June, 11–15.

14. Morris, H. (1976) Thomas Szasz and the manufacture of madness. In: H. Morris *On Guilt and Innocence*, p. 70. Berkeley: University of California Press.

15. Helzer, J. E., Clayton, P. J., Pambakian, R., Reich, T., Woodruff, R. A. Jr and Reveley, M. A. (1977) Reliability of psychiatric diagnoses. *Archives of General Psychiatry*, **34**, 136–41; Helzer, J. E., Robins, L. N., Taibleson, M., Woodruff, R. A. Jr, Reich, T. and Wish, E. D. (1977) Reliability of psychiatric diagnosis. I. A methodological review. *Archives of General Psychiatry*, **34**, 129–33; Spitzer, R. L., Forman, J. B. W. and Nee, J. (1979) DSM-III field trails. I. Initial interrater diagnostic reliability. *American Journal of Psychiatry*, **136**, 815–17; Grove, W. M., Andreasen, N. C., McDonald-Scott, P., Keller,

M. B. and Shapero, R. W. (1981) Reliability studies of psychiatric diagnosis. *Archives of General Psychiatry*, **38**, 408–13; Helzer, J. E., Brockington, I. F. and Kendell, R. E. (1981) Predictive validity of DSM-III and Feighner definitions of schizophrenia. *Archives of General Psychiatry*, **38**, 791–7.

16. Acheson, R. M. (1960) Observer error and variation in the interpretation of electrocardiograms in an epidemiological study of coronary heart disease. *British Journal of Preventive and Social Medicine*, **14**, 99–122.

17. Norden, C., Phillips, E., Levy, P. and Kass, E. (1970) Variation in interpretation of intravenous pyelograms. *American Journal of Epidemiology*, **91**, 155–60.

18. Felson, B., Morgan, W. K. C., Bristol, L. J., Pendergrass, E. P., Dessen, E. L., Linton, O. W. and Reger, R. B. (1973) Observations on the results of multiple readings of chest films in coal miners' pneumoconiosis. *Radiology*, **109**, 19–23.

19. Joint report of the Royal College of Physicians and the Royal College of Pathologists (1982) Medical aspects of death certification. *Journal of the Royal College of Physicians of London*, **16**, 206–18 (p. 213).

20. Koran, L. M. (1975) The reliability of clinical methods, data and judgments. *New England Journal of Medicine*, **293**, 642–6 (part I) and 695–701 (part II) (p. 700).

21. Steadman, H. J. and Cocozza, J. J. (1975) We can't predict who is dangerous. *Psychology Today* [January], 32–5 and 84; Diamond, B. L. (1974) The psychiatric prediction of dangerousness. *University of Pennsylvania Law Review*, **123**, 439–52.

22. *Baxtrom v. Herold*, 383 US 107 (1966).

23. Pollock, H. M. (1938) Is the paroled patient a menace to the community? *Psychiatric Quarterly*, **12**, 236–44; Cohen, L. H. and Freeman, H. (1945) How dangerous to the community are state hospital patients? *Connecticut State Medical Journal*, **9**, 697–9; Hastings, D. W. (1958) Follow-up results in psychiatric illness. *American Journal of Psychiatry*, **144**, 1057–66; Guze, S. B., Goodwin, D. W. and Crane, J. B. (1969) Criminality and psychiatric disorders. *Archives of General Psychiatry*, **20**, 583–91.

24. Zitrin, A., Hardesty, A. S., Burdock, E. I. and Drossman, A. K. (1976) Crime and violence among mental patients. *American Journal of Psychiatry*, **133**, 142–9; Lagos, J. M., Perlmutter, K. and Saexinger, H. (1977) Fear of the mentally ill: empirical support for the common man's response. *American Journal of Psychiatry*, **134**, 1134–7; Berger, P. A. and Gulevich, G. D. (1981) Violence and mental illness. In: D. A. Hamburg and M. B. Trudeau (eds.) *Biobehavioural Aspects of Aggression*. New York: Alan Liss Inc.

25. Steadman, H. J., Melick, M. E. and Cocozza, J. J. (1977) Arrest rates of persons released from New York State Department of Mental Hygiene psychiatric centers. Albany, NY: Division of Research, New York State Department of Mental Hygiene, unpublished manuscript; Rabkin, J. G. (1979) Criminal behaviour of discharged mental patients: a critical appraisal of the research. *Psychological Bulletin*, **86**, 1–27; Sosowsky, L. (1980) Explaining the increased arrest rate among mental patients: a cautionary note. *American Journal of Psychiatry*, **137**, 1602–5.

26. Yesavage, J. A., Werner, P. D., Becker, J. M. T. and Mills, M. J. (1982) The context of involuntary commitment on the basis of danger to others. *Journal of Nervous and Mental Disease*, **170**, 622–7.

27. Rofman, E. S., Askinazi, C. and Fant, E. (1980) The prediction of dangerous behavior in emergency civil commitment. *American Journal of Psychiatry*, **137**, 1061–4.

28. Monahan, J. (1981) *The Clinical Prediction of Violent Behaviors*. Rockville, Maryland: US Department of Health and Human Services (No. ADM, 81–921); Kroll, J. L. and Mackenzie, T. B. (1983) When psychiatrists are liable: risk management and violent patients. *Hospital and Community Psychiatry*, **34**, 29–37; Monahan, J. (1984) The

prediction of violent behaviour: toward a second generation of theory and policy. *American Journal of Psychiatry*, **141**, 10–15.

29. Roth, M. (1976) Schizophrenia and the theories of Thomas Szasz. *British Journal of Psychiatry*, **129**, 317–26.

29a. Felix: *Life of St Guthlac*, ed. B. Colgrave, pp. 127–9. Cambridge: Cambridge University Press, 1956.

30. Drew, K. F. (trans.) (1973) *The Lombard Laws*. Philadelphia: University of Pennsylvania Press.

31. *The Procheiros Nomos* (published by the Emperor Basil I at Constantinople between AD 867 and 879), trans. E. H. Freshfield. Cambridge: Cambridge University Press, 1928.

32. Bracton, H. (1256) *De Legibus et Consuetudinibus Angliae* (The Chronicles and Memorial of Great Britain and Ireland During the Middle Ages). London: Longman and Company, 1883.

33. Westman, B. H. (1974) The peasant family and crime in fourteenth-century England. *Journal of British Studies*, **13**, 1–18. See also Neugebauer, R. (1978) Treatment of the mentally ill in medieval and early modern England: a reappraisal. *Journal of the History of the Behavioral Sciences*, **14**, 158–69; and Neugebauer, R. (1979) Medieval and early modern theories of mental illness. *Archives of General Psychiatry*, **36**, 477–83.

34. *Wall Street Journal*, 17 August 1982.

35. Morse, S. J. (1982) Failed explanations and criminal responsibility: experts and the unconscious. *Virginia Law Review*, **68**, 971–1084.

36. AMA Committee on Medicolegal Problems (1984) Insanity defense in criminal trials and limitations of psychiatric testimony. *Journal of the American Medical Association*, **251**, 2967–81 (p. 2981).

37. Kadish, S. H. (1968) The decline of innocence. *Cambridge Law Journal*, **26**, 273–90. (p. 278).

37a. Report of the Committee on Mentally Abnormal Offenders (Chairman Lord Butler) 1975. Cmnd 6244. London: HMSO.

38. Morse, S. J. (1982) *Op. cit.*, p. 982, n. 34.

39. Feinberg, J. (1970) What is so special about mental illness? In: J. Feinberg *Doing and Deserving: Essays in the Theory of Responsibility*. Princeton: Princeton University Press.

40. Morris, H. (1976) Thomas Szasz and *The Manufacture of Madness*. In: H. Morris (ed.) *On Guilt and Innocence*. Berkeley: University of California Press.

41. Morris, H. (1976) *On Guilt and Innocence*. Berkeley: University of California Press.

42. Kadish, S. H. (1968) *Op. cit.*, p. 284, n. 35.

43. Feinberg, J. (1970) *Op. cit.*, p. 273.

44. Stone, A. (1982) The insanity defense on trial. *Harvard Law School Bulletin*, **33**, 15–21.

45. Waelder, R. (1952) Psychiatry and the problem of criminal responsibility. *University of Pennsylvania Law Review*, **101**, 378–90.

46. Devlin, P. (1959) *The Enforcement of Morals*, p. 17. London: Oxford University Press.

47. Wootton, B. (1963) The law, the doctor, and the deviant. *British Medical Journal*, ii, 197–202.

48. Lunn, V. (1985) The Danish experience: one model of psychiatric testimony to courts of law. In *Psychiatry, Human Rights and the Law*, ed. M. Roth & R. Bluglass, pp. 215–27. Cambridge University Press.

49. Roth, M. & Bluglass, R. (1985) *Psychiatry, Human Rights and the Law*. Cambridge University Press.

50. Penrose, L. S. (1939) Mental disease and crime: outline of a comparative study of European statistics. *British Journal of Medical Psychology*, **18**, 1–15.